THE TRANSFORMING POWER OF FASTING AND PRAYER

Personal Accounts of Spiritual Renewal

Bill Bright

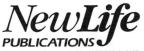

NewLife
PUBLICATIONS
A MINISTRY OF CAMPUS CRUSADE FOR CHRIST

The Transforming Power of Fasting & Prayer
Published by
NewLife Publications
A ministry of Campus Crusade for Christ
P. O. Box 593684
Orlando, FL 32859-3684

Design and typesetting by Genesis Publications.

Cover by David Marty Design.

Printed in the United States of America.

Library of Congress Cataloging-in-Publication Data
Bright, Bill.
    The transforming power of fasting & prayer : personal accounts of
    spiritual renewal / Bill Bright : foreword by Bill McCartney.
        p.   cm.
    Includes bibliographical references.
    ISBN 1-56399-090-3
    1. Fasting—Case studies.   2. Prayer—Christianity—Case studies.
  3. Evangelicalism. 4. Church renewal. I. Title.
    BV5055.B75   1997
    248.4'7—dc21   97-16983
                     CIP

Unless otherwise indicated, Scripture quotations are from the *New International Version,* © 1973, 1978, 1984 by the International Bible Society. Published by Zondervan Bible Publishers, Grand Rapids, Michigan.

Scripture quotations designated TLB are from *The Living Bible,* © 1971 by Tyndale House Publishers, Wheaton, Illinois.

Scripture quotations designated Amplified are from *The Amplified Bible,* © 1987 by The Zondervan Corporation, Grand Rapids, Michigan, and the Lockman Foundation, La Habra, California.

Scripture quotations designated NKJ are from the *New King James* version, © 1979, 1980, 1982 by Thomas Nelson Inc., Publishers, Nashville, Tennessee.

Scripture quotations designated NASB are from *The New American Standard Bible,* © 1960, 1962, 1963, 1968, 1971, 1972, 1973, 1975, 1977 by the Lockman Foundation, La Habra, California.

For more information, write:
L.I.F.E., Campus Crusade for Christ—P. O. Box 40, Flemmington Markets, 2129, Australia
Campus Crusade for Christ of Canada—Box 300, Vancouver, B.C., V6C 2X3, Canada
Campus Crusade for Christ—Fairgate House, King's Road, Tyseley, Birmingham, B11 2AA, England
Lay Institute for Evangelism, Campus Crusade for Christ—P. O. Box 8786, Auckland, New Zealand
Campus Crusade for Christ—Alexandra, P. O. Box 0205, Singapore 9115, Singapore
Great Commission Movement of Nigeria—P. O. Box 500, Jos, Plateau State, Nigeria, West Africa
Campus Crusade for Christ International—100 Sunport Lane, Orlando, FL 32809, USA

The Transforming Power of Fasting & Prayer *is a book of personal accounts of extended fasting and prayer, written from a spiritual perspective to encourage the body of Christ.*

The author is not a medical doctor, and it is not the purpose of this book to address in depth the physical or medical aspects of fasting. Most people can fast for forty days without complications if they follow guidelines. However, there are some people for whom a fast, because of medical conditions, would not be safe. Please take the necessary precautions and responsibility for your health, including consulting with a physician.

*Extended "water-only" fasts are **not** endorsed by this author. For both physical and spiritual reasons, it is advised that shorter fasts be completed prior to attempting an extended fast. Care in breaking a fast is critical and should be done slowly with extreme caution. I advise you to act responsibly as you undertake fasting, and seek God's guidance concerning an extended fast.*

For additional information on how to fast, refer to The Coming Revival, 7 Basic Steps to Successful Fasting & Prayer, *and the Appendices in this book.*

Dedication

During my first forty-day fast in 1994, the Lord gave me the assurance that He was going to send a great spiritual revival to His Church. This sovereign move of God would be followed by the greatest spiritual harvest in the history of the Church. However, with that assurance of the coming revival was the admonition that believers must meet the conditions of 2 Chronicles 7:14 before He would send the full measure of His Holy Spirit upon His people. Note the four conditions of this powerful promise:

> If my people, who are called by my name, will *humble themselves* and *pray* and *seek my face* and *turn from their wicked ways*, then will I hear from heaven and will forgive their sin and will heal their land.

Then, to my amazement, the Lord impressed me to pray for two million believers to join me in fasting and praying for forty days to help fulfill the conditions of that promise and to see the revival come to pass in our time.

As I explained in my book, *The Coming Revival: America's Call to Fast, Pray, and "Seek God's Face,"* I did not know of a single believer in North America who had fasted forty days when I began my fast. Naturally, I was deeply puzzled. How could I recruit two million to fast and pray when it was obvious that most Christians were unaware of the revolutionary power of fasting?

God's answer to my unspoken question was that He would call them to fast and pray as He had called me. My role was to fast and pray and to write an informative book that explains the "how to" of fasting and prayer. He would do the rest. That is one reason I wrote *The Coming Revival.*

7

Now I dedicate this second book on fasting to the two million courageous Christians—to each and every one of you—who obediently respond to God's call to spend forty days in fasting and prayer for national and worldwide revival and for the fulfillment of the Great Commission by the end of the year 2000.

Contents

Acknowledgments

Through the years, I have written many books and hundreds of articles. In the beginning of my ministry, I personally researched and wrote, and many times rewrote, each published piece. Today, my responsibilities of leading a large worldwide movement, along with an extensive travel schedule, no longer allow me that luxury. Therefore, I would like to acknowledge the efforts of all who contributed to this book.

Without the thousands of people who completed an extended fast and those who took the time to send me their testimony, *The Transforming Power of Fasting & Prayer* would not have been possible. My thanks to all of you and to God for working in each of your lives. Because of your efforts, this book will be an inspiration to millions of others throughout the world to seek God's face in fasting and prayer.

Along with your testimonies, many more people were involved in this effort. My special heartfelt thanks to writer/researcher Lydia DeLorenzo. My continual gratitude goes to the NewLife Publications staff: Dr. Joe Kilpatrick, Executive Director, who took the idea for this book and nurtured it along to a finished product; Michelle Treiber, printing; and Joette Whims, editing. My gratitude also goes to Lynn Copeland of Genesis Publications for typesetting and to Dr. William Nix for research and ideas.

Special thanks to Dick Eastman, Shirley Dobson, Carlton Pearson, Eddie and Alice Smith, Wesley Campbell, and Ronnie Floyd for their generous contributions of time and materials, and for their individual efforts to promote extended fasting and prayer.

Also, many of my associates in the President's Office have played major roles in helping me organize and lead three fasting and prayer gatherings. The first was held in Orlando in 1994, the second in Los Angeles in 1995, and the third in St. Louis in 1996. I am deeply indebted to Sid Wright, my Chief of Staff and Coordinator for the fasting and prayer gatherings. Matt Anderson, Mary Graham, John Rogers, Randy Murphy, Paula Marolis, and many others also helped make these gatherings possible.

Special recognition and appreciation goes to Sir John Templeton and his selection committee who chose me for the 1996 Templeton Prize for the Advancement of Religion. The money I received from this international award (more than one million dollars) is being used in its entirety to encourage fasting and prayer around the world.

Finally, I save my dearest expressions of appreciation for my beloved wife, Vonette, who has encouraged me through three forty-day fasts in the last three years and co-chairs with me the national fasting and prayer gatherings.

Foreword

When I embarked on my forty-day fast in January 1996, my primary motive was a deep, desperate longing to draw closer to God; I hungered continually for greater intimacy with the Lord. Scripture tells us that fasting allows us to dwell with the Lord in the posture most pleasing to Him by intensifying in our hearts and bodies the qualities of humility, brokenness, and contrition. I realized then I was walking a path that very few Christians had tread before me.

A strong secondary focus of my fast, however, was to pray for the outcome of the Promise Keepers Men's Clergy Conference in Atlanta (February 13–15, 1996). Because pastors play such a critical role in guiding the Church toward biblical harmony in this day of denominational divisiveness and spiritual mediocrity, I began pleading daily that God would pour out His Spirit in Atlanta, bringing unity and refreshment to His shepherds. Everything I'd read and heard from the field confirmed that our pastors were an increasingly beleaguered, burned-out bunch who, because of unrealistic pressure and expectations from their congregations, were falling in record numbers into sin and even leaving their life's calling.

While I have made it a practice over the past twenty years to fast for part of two days each week (after the example of John Wesley), I had never before considered anything approaching a forty-day fast. However, my burning desire was to draw near to God, to be cleansed of impurity, and to be fashioned into a tool God could use. For all intents and purposes, the fast proceeded smoothly. I lost a lot of weight and experienced incomparably sweet times of fellowship with the Lord. I felt as if God affected a deep work of inner purification within me. Yet, as I neared the end of the fast, I began to sense great turbulence in my heart. I realized that I was struggling with the question, "What is my true motivation for fasting?" Was it pride or *achievement* (typical of an ex-football coach)? Ironically, a breakthrough came at day 39. I came across John 4:34 in which Jesus tells His disciples, "My food is to do the will of him who sent me and to finish his work."

Suddenly, I understood what Jesus meant, and at that moment I gained a new perspective on fasting. Jesus was explaining that what He practiced and modeled to His disciples is what God also requires of us. Like our Lord, when we fast, our *food* is "to do the will of Him who sent me." My fast was almost over, but I had finally discovered how to fast with a right heart toward God. So few Christians realize how healthy it is to say "no" to one's physical needs and "yes" to our spiritual hunger.

The Clergy Conference was, by any measure, a powerful event. During our three days together, God's Spirit descended on the approximately 40,000 pastors in attendance from across the world. Thousands of us left renewed, inspired, and, in many cases, released from the competitive striving that cripples our Christian witness to the world.

But something else amazing happened in connection with the Clergy Conference: sensing its importance, tens of thousands of men and women across the globe prayed and fasted for the event. What could possibly please God more than for His Church to *sacrifice* to know Him and see Him move?

In his book *The Coming Revival*, Bill Bright paints a striking picture, challenging two million Christians to undertake a personal forty-day fast by the end of the year 2000. In so doing, he suggests, Christians willing to sacrifice at this level will be instrumental in igniting a spiritual awakening across our land and throughout the world unlike any other in our lifetime.

Clearly, God is planting seeds of revival throughout His Church. For instance, on October 4, 1997, in Washington, D.C., Promise Keepers will host an event called *Stand in the Gap: A Sacred Assembly of Men.* In obedience to God's invitation to His people to stand up for truth and righteousness (Ezekiel 22:30 and Joel 2:15), a multitude of men will gather in our nation's capitol to humble themselves before God, kneel to confess their sins, and repent for their failure as Christians to stand in the gap for this nation. They will plead for God's mercy on our land. In preparation for the event, men and women will fast and pray, and begin to earnestly embrace a lifestyle of true repentance, that is, a lifestyle of "turning away from sin." I believe *Stand in the Gap* is one of many means God will use to administer an electroshock to America's slumbering Church.

Presently, there are countless prayer and fasting movements erupting across the landscape. By God's sovereign prompting, individuals, churches, and even cities are catching the vision and holding sacred forty-day fasts. New networks are forming every week of pastors committed to fasting for the Church and their communities.

In this shared activity, we are seeing denominational walls beginning to fall and racial and cultural divisions being dissolved. People who previously would have nothing to do with one another are now, through this binding call to fast and pray for common causes, experiencing a spiritual unity unseen in this century.

Similar movements are occurring internationally. In Korea and throughout Asia and Europe, indeed on every continent and in many countries, people are coming together for the singular purpose of fasting and prayer that they might discern God's will for their families, communities, and nations. As Dr. Bright said in *The Coming Revival,* this work of God is exploding "like dynamite."

Brothers and sisters, *God is up to something!* He is calling His people into deeper waters. Are we ready to respond? Are we on high alert? Are Christian men and women really determined in their hearts, minds, and bodies to be the genuine "people of God"?

Do we desire, by whatever means necessary, to be salt and light to a dark and rotting culture, to obey when God calls us to fast and pray for our nation? It is an incomparable calling, but Christ has appointed us as His royal priesthood (1 Peter 2:9), anointed and equipped for such duties, if we will only believe and obey.

Read these pages, then let your heart be filled with hope. We serve an awesome God who longs to involve us in His plans. He is up to something. *Get ready, Church!*

Coach Bill McCartney
Founder/CEO, Promise Keepers

Preface

In *The Coming Revival: America's Call to Fast, Pray, and "Seek God's Face,"* the Lord led me to sound the call for two million believers to fast and pray for forty days for national and worldwide revival and the fulfillment of the Great Commission. At that time in 1994, I wondered, *Would Christians of the 1990s complete an extended fast? Would they humble themselves and seek God's face, repenting for the sins of America and praying for revival? Am I absolutely certain that when two million believers fast and pray for revival for forty days, the Lord will respond with an unprecedented outpouring of revival in answer to their faith and discipline?* The Lord assured me that He would speak to His people.

Since then, in our radio broadcasts, speaking engagements, magazine articles, through Campus Crusade for Christ staff members and our many friends around the world, my staff and I have asked people to let us know if they are among the two million whom God has called to fast for revival. "Could you tell us some of the changes or impressions you experienced, both during the fast and afterward?" we asked. In addition, we requested permission to publish their letters to encourage and bless others.

Letters, faxes, and E-mail notes have poured in from Christians across America and around the world who have completed an extended fast. While the two million are still being led by the Holy Spirit to join us, it is clear that revival has already begun across America. An amazing awakening is taking place on scores of college campuses. Thousands of churches are shaking off their "standard operating procedures" and allowing the Holy Spirit to cleanse, restore, and renew.

If you have ever doubted that God works among His people today, prepare to have your mind changed and your faith dramatically expanded. The fasting testimonies that I have received are filled with renewed faith and a special portrayal of God's mercy and abundant love. I have been repeatedly moved and uplifted by these messages of answered prayers for spiritual growth, salvation for unsaved friends and family, physical healing, financial needs, release from sin, specific guidance, and a greater devotion to serve the Lord. Marriages have been restored, campuses awakened, and churches revived. God's power is indeed being poured out upon His people as a result of extended fasts to "seek God's face."

As you read these personal accounts, you will observe that the Spirit of the Lord has become very real to those who have yielded to His call to fast and pray for spiritual revival. As a result, some have gone on to ignite a fire in their church or community, which has in turn brought about local fasting conferences across the country! The blessing of the fast does not fade after the forty days, but the deeper intimacy that develops in a Christian's relationship with the Lord continues to bless in a profound way.

Following my forty-day fast in 1994, more than 600 Christian leaders joined me in Orlando, Florida, to fast and pray for national and world revival and the fulfillment of the Great Commission. In 1995, I was led to experience a second forty-day fast. A few months later, more than 3,500 Christian leaders met in Los Angeles in November 1995 to fast and pray. During my third forty-day fast, nearly 4,000 met at Fasting & Prayer '96 in St. Louis—and tens of thousands more across the country joined us by satellite transmission. In circles of ten, we knelt to repent, to worship, and to bring our petitions for revival to the Lord. We stood and glorified His name in song and thanksgiving. Speaker after speaker opened our hearts and minds to the work of the Lord and exhorted us to serve Him and Him alone. (Three of the messages from the St. Louis gathering are reprinted in the Appendices.)

It is with great anticipation that we prepare to join with pastors and other Christian leaders on November 12–14, 1997, at the Dallas/Fort Worth Airport's Hyatt Regency for Fasting & Prayer '97, a three-day gathering for the purpose of confessing our sins before God and praying for healing and revival. Because of the potential impact of Fasting & Prayer '97, both personally and on our nation, we are helping to establish as many as 10,000 satellite down-link sites across America so that millions will be able to participate in their own communities. Thousands of churches nationwide will be able to take part in this unique opportunity. As hundreds of thousands, perhaps millions, gather in unified prayer, I can only imagine how God will respond when so many of His people humbly seek His face. I believe we will experience a mighty visitation of God as we acknowledge and repent of the sin that entangles and encounter the One who forgives.

My heart leaps with joy over the reports of unprecedented spiritual blessing experienced by thousands of Christians as they heed God's call to fast and pray for personal, national, and worldwide revival. Here are just a few of the thrilling accounts:

- Forty pastors in Spokane, Washington, joined together in a forty-day fast.
- More than ninety churches in Bakersfield, California, fasted forty days through Lent.
- One hundred twenty pastors in the Dallas, Texas, area have just completed a forty-day fast.
- Eighty-three churches in the United Kingdom are participating in extended fasts.

And these are only the tip of God's spiritual iceberg. Truly He is building a movement of fasting and prayer that is sweeping this nation and the world!

As we humble ourselves, pray, seek God's face, and turn from our evil ways, He will do great and mighty, even supernatural, things among us. If you are one of the "two million," but haven't written in yet, I look forward to reading *your* fasting testimony. To all of you who have joined with me in seeking God's face in this way, I want to express my deepest love and to give Him all the praise.

In spite of our personal and national sin, I am confident that God wants to spare our nation and send a great spiritual awakening to North America and the world before the end of the year 2000. Believers everywhere must catch the vision. Will you answer God's call to action? Will you join with thousands of other Christians in seeking God's face and power to change your life, our nation, and the world?

Perhaps you have felt the Holy Spirit call you to a forty-day fast, but are hesitant to begin. If so, let these moving testimonies act as evidence that people just like you—many of whom had never fasted before—have accomplished what they felt was impossible. My prayer is that these exciting accounts will be the encouragement you need to take the next step.

CHAPTER 1

Fasting, Prayer, and the Great Commission

If my people, who are called by my name, will humble themselves and pray and seek my face and turn from their wicked ways, then will I hear from heaven and will forgive their sin and will heal their land.

—2 CHRONICLES 7:14

Throughout my walk with the Lord these past fifty years, He has blessed me with a marvelous family, a dynamic ministry that keeps growing for His glory, and a staff that is greater than all the words I could possibly write. He has showered me with so many good things that it is beyond my ability to adequately respond. Certainly among them is the more than one-million-dollar Templeton Prize, which I received at the hands of Prince Philip and Sir John Templeton in Buckingham Palace in May 1996.

Even before I received the prize, our Lord definitely led me to designate it for fasting and prayer. All of the proceeds from the Templeton Prize have been assigned to encourage and equip millions of Christians around the world to join us in fasting and praying for world revival. Using those funds to emphasize spiritual renewal through fasting with prayer will do more to help fulfill the Great Commission—to introduce large numbers of people to

Christ and disciple them to win and disciple others—than any other investment we could make.

After forty-five years of emphasizing evangelism, discipleship, and fulfillment of the Great Commission, some may think that I have gone off on a tangent with my strong emphasis on fasting and prayer. The fact is that the best way to help individuals become evangelists for Christ is to bring them into a relationship with God in which the Holy Spirit renews them. Only fasting meets the criteria of each aspect of 2 Chronicles 7:14. When you humble yourself and pray and seek God's face and turn from your wicked ways, something happens to you and you get excited about the Lord in a way that you do not through any other means.

Why fasting?

First, Christians who fast say that it sharpens and sensitizes their spiritual faculties to become more in tune with what God is doing throughout the world. As you read the firsthand accounts of their experiences, be encouraged to seek God's power in your life, your family, your church, and the nation. God is waiting to bless and use you in unprecedented ways as you respond to His prompting to make fasting and prayer a vital part of your life.

Second, fasting results in a greater intimacy with and a deeper enthusiasm for God, which in turn spills over into every other area of life. The joy of the Lord becomes much more visible to others, and the motivation to witness is greater. Fasting and prayer will do more to prepare millions throughout the world for revival than anything else we can do. In addition, because God honors fasting and prayer, more people will come to Jesus Christ in the sweep of that renewal.

Third, fasting prepares us for a spiritual harvest. Today, people throughout the world are hungry for the gospel. I have been a believer since 1944, and I can assure you that God is doing a great and powerful work, unprecedented in this century. This is most definitely a remarkable time of harvest. Doors of opportunity are quickly opening all over the world, and God's people are responding to the call in great numbers. More people are hearing the gospel and coming to know the Lord today than ever before in the history of the human race!

Unfortunately, Scripture assures us, and history also confirms, that this harvest is not going to last long. In the natural world, ripened fruit must be harvested within a certain span of time—two or three weeks at most—before it falls to the ground and decays. The same is true for the harvest of grain. In a similar way, the spiritual harvest we are seeing today will last only a few strategic years. However, I believe we will see more people come to Christ before the end of the year 2000 than we have seen in two thousand years of evangelism.

Perhaps you have fasted without even one word of encouragement from the closest Christians around you. Let these personal accounts confirm that you are not alone— there are thousands of others who are fasting!

If you are a minister uncertain whether your congregation will respond to the call, read about churches which have never before fasted that now regularly host fasting and prayer meetings. Many pastors write that they have found a new spiritual depth and passion in themselves and their congregations.

If you are wondering if your community could be changed by fasting and prayer, take heart in the many examples of citywide fasts, such as the one in Houston, Texas.

All of these personal accounts—and many more that wouldn't fit in these pages—are endorsements of the Lord's readiness to respond to us when we seek His face in fasting and prayer. Are you longing for more of God and less of yourself? Are you willing to open your heart and mind to His call to fast and pray for personal revival that revolutionizes our churches and cities, and results in a revival in our beloved country? Will America once again believe "In God We Trust"? Will the scales of justice be grounded in biblical truth? Will the outcry of the Church in this nation force the long-standing evils of prejudice and greed to be exposed and eradicated?

I fully expect that the Great Commission will be fulfilled in my lifetime. As God's people get right with Him through fasting with prayer and become motivated to seek the lost for Christ—to change their homes, their churches, schools, and local governments—I am sure God will honor those efforts. He *will* hear from heaven, forgive our sin, and heal our land as He promised.

CHAPTER 2

Fasting Transforms Us to Transform the World

I can't fast even *one* day," a young person lamented not long ago. "How could I possibly fast for forty days?" For most of us (including myself when God first impressed upon me to fast for forty days), an extended fast seems so unattainable, so *impossible* to do. But we can step out in faith (even with doubts)and say: "Lord, if this is what you want me to do, with Your help I'll begin. I'll take it day by day and humble myself before You to listen to You. I desire *You*, Lord, above all else." When we surrender to God in faith, He enables us to do everything He calls us to do.

People occasionally ask me, "What is the importance of the number 40 in fasting?" In the Bible, God seems to give special recognition to the number 40. Often it is the number of complete testing and repentance. Consider these examples from Scripture:

- The flood lasted for forty days upon the earth (Genesis 7:17).

- Moses sojourned in Midian for forty years before God appeared to him in a burning bush (Acts 7:29,30).

- The Israelites were delivered into the hands of the Philistines for forty years (Judges 13:1).

- Moses was on Mount Sinai for forty days and nights (Exodus 34:28).

- The Israelites wandered in the desert for forty years (Deuteronomy 8:2).

- Goliath defied Israel for forty days (1 Samuel 17:16).
- Due to the Pharaoh's pride, Egypt was made desolate for forty years (Ezekiel 29:12).
- Jonah warned Nineveh to repent or be destroyed in forty days (Jonah 3:4).
- Jesus fasted forty days and nights during His temptation (Matthew 4:2).
- Jesus appeared after the resurrection for a period of forty days (Acts 1:3).

Let me emphasize, however, that it is not the number of days you fast that is important—except for the fact that for most of us forty days is a big commitment, a huge effort, and an amazing achievement. In my case, it took forty days for God to show me all He wanted to do, to break down strongholds I was unaware of, and to open my heart to fuller obedience. It is not the number of days that magically "summons" God to us. Fasting helps us tear down the box we've put Him in—as well as the box we have put ourselves in—thereby helping us find new ways to worship Him and submit to Him on a higher level.

How Will God Change Me?

Fasting forces us to depend solely on God. C. S. Lewis wrote in his book *Letters to an American Lady:*

> It is a dreadful truth that the state of (as you say) 'having to depend solely on God' is what we all dread most. And of course that just shows how very much, how almost exclusively, we have been depending on things. But trouble goes so far back in our lives and is now so deeply ingrained, we *will* not turn to Him as long as He leaves us anything else to turn to...Perhaps when those moments come, they will feel happiest who have been forced (however unwittingly) to begin practicing it here on earth. It is good of Him to *force* us; but dear me, how hard to *feel* that it is good at the time.[1]

When we fast, we turn from the "things" that daily grab our attention and focus deeply on Him. During that time, we come to realize how much food and the things of this world are occupying our thoughts, time, activities, and finances. Some may realize, too, that they have been famished for spiritual food!

Could it be that you are surviving spiritually on bread and water? Are you willing to boldly turn from human interests and pleasures for a time? Of course, there may be nothing wrong with the television shows we watch, magazines we read, shopping, sports, or even the myriad of church social activities that occupy our time. The point is, are we willing to lay them down for forty days and focus on our loving Redeemer, our Protector and Provider, our Lord and King?

Perhaps you do not fast because you fear that you will harm your body. (For information of fasting's physical effects, see Appendix D, "Physical Aspects of Fasting.") If you have not fasted before, start by fasting one meal, then one day a week, then three days, then work up to ten days. See if your apprehensions diminish. Reading these testimonies of others who have fasted for forty days will also help shrink your fears. Thousands of others, just like you, have completed what they once thought was impossible. However, that still may not mean you should attempt a forty-day fast if God has not called you to it. He may not be calling you to fast at this time, but be open to His leading. All of us are biblically called to fast. Jesus said "when you fast," not "if you fast" (Matthew 6:16). Let the Spirit guide you with the details.

As we fast, God will show us the areas in our lives that we keep off limits to Him and the ways we seek to control our lives rather than let Him lead us. Any coldness in our hearts melts during a fast, and we become transformed and empowered to walk in His ways.

Will God Answer My Prayer?

If I fast, will my prayer be answered? Scripture gives us numerous examples of how God responds to His people when they fast. When the people of Nineveh realized that the Lord would judge their city by destroying it, they humbled themselves in fear and fasted, and God preserved them. Esther and all of her people fasted before the Lord for protection when the king was deceived into signing a decree to destroy them. God protected Esther's people, and the king changed his decree.

However, God doesn't always release us from our trials. Before His trial and crucifixion, Jesus prayed, "Father, if you are willing, take this cup from me; yet not my will, but yours be done" (Luke 22:42).

> *Fasting, as a purifying discipline, helps us draw closer to Him and surrender our will to His ways.*

God allowed Jesus to suffer and die for us. Christ's death and resurrection allow us to have access to the Father and to receive eternal salvation. God is a good and loving Father who hears and answers us. He wants to abundantly give us what is best for us. However, He knows what we do not know. His ways are higher than our ways. In that same passage in Luke, we read, "An angel from heaven appeared to [Jesus] and strengthened him" (v. 43). God gave Jesus strength to endure the suffering. God also may not give you what you want, but He will give you what you need. Fasting, as a purifying discipline, helps us draw closer to Him and surrender our will to His ways.

Can a fast coerce God into giving us what we want? If that is our motive, we are not humbling ourselves. Fasting without recognizing God's sovereign control and Lordship is, at the least, empty. In Isaiah 58:3,4, God gives a solemn warning about fasting for ourselves and not to the Lord:

"Why have we fasted," they say, "and you have not seen it? Why have we humbled ourselves, and you have not noticed?" Yet on the day of your fasting, you do as you please and exploit all your workers. Your fasting ends in quarreling and strife...You cannot fast as you do today and expect your voice to be heard on high.

Examining your motives and actions prior to and during your fast will keep you from sinning against the Lord. First, ask yourself if you have repented of all known sin. Second, practice Spiritual Breathing—confessing your sin as it occurs and praying to be filled with the Holy Spirit—to keep your fasting motive pure before the Lord. Third, I suggest that you keep a notebook handy during your fast to record the areas of your life that need to change as God reveals them to you through His Spirit and His Word. Implement those changes in the way He leads you.

Fasting is a means to answered prayer; God will answer your prayers according to His grace. But more than that, you will become more like Jesus, be renewed, and in turn, be constrained by the love of Christ to help reach the world for Him.

Should I Tell Others That I Am Fasting?

Many people are reluctant to tell others that they are fasting so they will avoid the sin that the Pharisees committed—fasting just to gain recognition. I strongly believe, however, that it is a trick of the enemy to keep our fasting a secret. By isolating ourselves from the support of other Christians, we may be more susceptible to doubts and negative influences (both human and demonic). We need the prayer shield of our Christian friends and family members to help us continue when we feel alone and when the enemy tempts us to give up.

People are bound to notice that you are not eating. However, I have found that unless you see them daily, they do not consider your skipped meal of much concern. If you are asked, nonbelievers may be satisfied by a brief answer such as, "I have other plans for lunch today." Christians should be satisfied when you answer that you are fasting today. If friends and family express concern for your health, ease their fears by telling them that you will stop fasting the moment you feel you are harming your body or if the Lord leads you to end your fast. When Christians express a genuine interest in fasting for spiritual reasons, the door is open for you to talk about how fasting contributes to answered prayer and personal and worldwide revival.

On the other hand, there is usually no good purpose for telling strangers or casual acquaintances that you are completing a forty-day fast. Often they will subject you to a lot of questions that you may not want to answer. Some may jump to the conclusion that you are a fanatic or part of a New Age group. In any case, use your best judgment and the Lord's leading in telling people about your fast.

Listening to the Lord

While fasting, dedicate as much time as possible to communing with the Lord. It is unwise to fast unless you can arrange your schedule to spend special time with the Lord each day. For some it may be necessary to maintain a busy schedule during a fast. While this is not ideal, the Lord honors the heart that seeks and serves Him. Whenever possible, clear your daily schedule of any optional activities. Use meal times to worship the Lord and wait on Him. Pray during the night hours if the Lord awakens you. These quiet, undistracted times can open the way for you to hear His voice in a special way.

A person usually has greater clarity during a fast, and sees spiritual needs and comprehends God's Word on a deeper level. As we make extra time for God by meditating on Bible passages, reading other inspiring materials, and opening ourselves to more intimate communion with

Him throughout the day, a richer experience in prayer will begin to permeate our thoughts.

Remorse may grip your heart for the sins of the world and for the tremendous suffering inflicted on others because of war, crime, greed, and evil. You may find yourself in tears over these atrocities, begging God to forgive us our long-standing sins as a country and interceding for those in great need throughout the world. Often we are drawn into deeper prayer by a greater realization that each day many in this world are dying without knowing Christ and many more have yet to turn to Him. As we humble ourselves before God, our prayers often become more impassioned for the lost and for those who minister as pastors, missionaries, teachers, and evangelists.

So many of those who have submitted fasting testimonies joyfully describe a deeper closeness to our Lord while fasting than they had ever experienced before. They described a nearness of His presence in all of their thoughts and desires. It is a sacred time. Yet you should know that others who undergo a forty-day fast in true humility and repentance deeply seeking God's face do *not* have a

> *So many of those who have submitted fasting testimonies joyfully describe a deeper closeness to our Lord while fasting than they had ever experienced before.*

"mountaintop experience." Some report no particular results at all. For others, their fast was physically, emotionally, and spiritually grueling, but they knew they had been called by God to fast, and they completed it unto Him as an act of worship.

I believe the Lord is especially honored by those who are faithful when no light shines through. The apostle Thomas needed to see and touch the hands and side of Jesus before he would believe in Christ's resurrection.

Our Lord gave Thomas the proof he needed to believe, but said, "Because you have seen me, you have believed; blessed are those who have not seen and yet have believed" (John 20:29). When we fast unto the Lord, we leave the results in His capable hands and trust in His Fatherly goodness and love.

Most people who undergo an extended fast do see God work in their lives in a new, rich way. As you read the life-changing stories that follow, you will see again and again God's kindness and grace at work among His people.

CHAPTER 3

Life-Changing Accounts

Through my many years of ministry, I have learned that God works in unique ways among His people. That is the case in fasting, too. Although Christians may have similar routines, emotions, and circumstances during a fast, each person will experience an individual communion with God. This also holds true for church-wide and citywide fasts. In each situation, God responds to the humble hearts of His people and moves according to His will. He answers prayer to satisfy the desires and needs of His children—and to glorify His name. These individual workings of God will be very evident in the life-changing accounts that follow.

Most of the testimonies are from individuals who have completed an extended fast on their own, many for forty days. The Lord, in turn, used many of these pioneers to encourage others to fast. As a result, churchwide fasts began, then citywide fasts[1]. National and worldwide efforts are now underway!

As I read each of these testimonies, tears of joy came to my eyes. Our Lord surely is moving among His Church in a deep and powerful way. He is using fasting and prayer to bring us closer to His heart and His will.

Each account touched me in a different way. I empathized with those who obtained God's power to bring them through an extended fast; I cried with those who recounted the sorrow of revealed sin and the joy of their own repentance and God's cleansing. And I rejoiced with those who saw dramatic answers to prayer through their fast.

When a "forty-day" or "extended" fast is mentioned, it refers to forty continuous days, drinking only fruit and vegetable juices, herbal teas, and water. Others chose to fast in the way they felt most capable. Those fasts ranged from one day per week for forty weeks, to two twenty-day fasts separated by a length of time, to continuous fasting up to forty days. Some completed a partial fast, such as a "Daniel" fast of plain vegetarian foods. Each Christian should follow his heart, the Lord's leading, and personal medical direction when undertaking an extended fast.

We have grouped these testimonies according to the scope of the fast—individual, churchwide, citywide, national, or international—not for any kind of ranking or earthly glory, but so that those of you who are interested in either fasting as an individual or initiating a corporate fast will have an easy reference. For the testimonies to come through with originality and spontaneity, our editors have made every effort to preserve the original content and have made only minor additions or corrections for clarity. Portions, rather than entire letters and interviews, are given.

> *This is what the coming revival will be all about—calling the people of God to repentance and bringing them back to their first love.*

I am often reminded of something I have tried to teach our Campus Crusade staff and others: All we really have to do as believers, from the time we get up in the morning until we go to bed at night, is to love God with all of our heart and soul and mind and strength, obey His commands, and trust His promises. That is all. Everything else is secondary.

This is what the coming revival will be all about—calling the people of God to repentance and bringing them back to their first love, to a life of faith and joyful obedience. These testimonies reveal the power of God to touch hearts through fasting and prayer, to enable us to live the abundant life through repentance and faith, and to bring personal—and, eventually, national—revival.

Much can be learned from all these accounts, for God is at work and a great revival is coming! See how these pioneers discovered a new intimacy with God and a revolutionary new power in daily living, in their witness for our Lord, and in answers to prayer. I encourage you to read the heartwarming testimonies that follow with an attitude of prayer, asking for God's guidance on how you, too, can have a closer walk with Him and can influence others to join you in surrendering all to Him.

I pray that their stories of personal renewal will inspire you to join them and millions more whom God has called and blessed through serious and extended fasting and prayer.

Individual Fasting and Prayer

No matter who we are or what kind of ministry God has given us, He still works through individuals. That is the beauty of the gospel message. God brings us into His family one by one and works with us individually to help us mature as His children. The same is true in how He works in our lives when we fast and pray. Paul writes in Philippians 2:13: "It is God who works in you to will and to act according to his good purpose." He meets our needs as individuals and answers our prayers in unique ways.

The testimonies in this section show the many ways God is working through fasting and prayer. Some Christians received miraculous answers to prayer; others saw their enthusiasm for fasting spread to friends; and some experienced changes in their ministry or received a new passion for serving God.

Many of the writers tell how God gave them the strength to maintain their fast for forty days. People were introduced to our Lord through answered prayers during fasting. As you read these testimonies, you will see how God is beginning to revive His people all over our country.

Although my staff and I received many more testimonies that were just as thrilling, we did not have room to print them all. These were chosen for variety so that the stories could touch the greatest amount of readers. We have not put these individual accounts in any particular order and have honored requests to omit last names or cities.

I encourage you to read through the experiences prayerfully, asking God to show you if He wants you to be part of the two million Christians we are inviting to join us in fasting. If you are not led to fast at this time, then ask God to give you a deeper sense of His presence in your prayer life and a greater commitment to helping fulfill the Great Commission. But no matter what your circumstances are or how He is leading you, expect Him to bless you through these inspiring accounts.

Bob

Many of those who fasted shared how they had received victory over trials. This testimony from Bob, a Florida pastor, shows the power of prayer and fasting in defeating Satan in the material realm.

I have just completed my forty-day fast and found it to be a powerful, renewing experience. It was a personal revival, and I believe the forty days of prayer and fasting have made a difference in myself, my family, my church, and my country. Satan worked, but Christ worked better, and I saw several miracles happen in my life during those days.

I grew up in an evangelical church, graduated from a church college and a seminary, and didn't ever recall hearing a sermon or reading a book on fasting. I had pastored for twenty years and rarely talked about it, and had not personally fasted for more than an occasional meal.

Even though I had not fasted much, I felt compelled to fast for forty days for my country, my church, and my family. It proved to be an unforgettable time of spiritual renewal. I noticed several amazing things happening. My prayer life took on a new intimacy with Christ. My preaching was more powerfully anointed by the Holy Spirit. I had more yearning in my heart for my people. They seemed to respond more openly during altar times. Somehow as I sacrificed my physical body, my spirit grew in holiness.

I knew I was on to something because Satan began to work. After the first week, he hit me where it hurts—my finances. Seventeen hundred dollars of unplanned expenses came up within just a few days. I decided Satan didn't like my fasting. But I was determined to continue.

The following Tuesday, the Lord provided. A man bought my antique car that had been for sale for over a year. That night in board meeting, the church board shocked me with a $5,000 raise for the year. I was $10,000 richer in just one day! I am not suggesting by this that fasting is a good way to make money. I am simply saying that our obedience in fasting somehow moves the hand of God to meet our needs and the needs of others.

~

If you and I are into works, then we are out of grace. If we are in grace, then we are out of works. Any time we get into works, the grace of God ceases to operate on our behalf. God has no choice but to back off and wait until we have finished trying to handle things ourselves.

—Joyce Meyer
If Not for the Grace of God

William

Like many who shared their testimony, William experienced an anointing of the Holy Spirit and a deep excitement through his fasting. He lives in Florida.

Forty days seemed like an awfully long time, but with a strong desire I purposed in my heart to do this. Another concern I had was my job, which involves a lot of strenuous labor. I am on my feet most of the day, sometimes lifting, sometimes climbing ladders, and I wondered whether I could fast that long and still do the job. Much to my amazement, I found that I had more strength, "get up and go," and motivation during the fast than when I was eating. I kept up a full schedule both day and night the entire forty days, which included preaching and teaching.

I discerned a definite increased anointing of the Holy Spirit as I spoke the Word of God. The spiritual intensity has continued with me even after the fast was over, even to this very time. My times of meditation in the Word were often phenomenal and glorious as the Scriptures would unfold before me. There was, it seemed, a greater sensitivity and intensity in prayer. The forty-day fast was much easier than I expected. I'm so glad I did it. I wouldn't trade it for the world. It was a definite life-changing time. I sense within me a deep excitement that I cannot explain.

I just spoke with a man in the congregation who has been separated from his wife for two years. Three weeks ago she was filing for divorce...But this week she called him (they had almost no communication for months) saying she wanted to make the marriage work and asking if he would take her back. Of course, he said yes. This is a miracle. It is a glorious answer to many, many prayers. Another couple in the church has also recently come together after a two-year separation. This is supernatural. It is the hand of God.

Since the fast, I have a deeper, clearer sense in my relationship with God, a submissiveness to the will of God, a willingness to yield to His initiations, a quietness, a contentment, a steadfastness, a commitment to His cross, and a resolve to follow Him wherever He leads.

ॐ

[Elijah] fasted forty days as he walked to Mt. Horeb...He left there under a mighty anointing of God and returned to Israel to execute the judgments of the Lord. Never again did he flee from man or woman. Faith so dominated his being that even death could not master him, and he was taken up by a chariot of fire into heaven.

—Gordon Lindsay
Prayer & Fasting: The Master Key to the Impossible

Robin

Robin, from Illinois, is director for the Christian Care Crisis Pregnancy Centers. She helped expand her church's emphasis on prayer to include fasting. Her own fasting has helped her to walk by faith.

I heard that Dr. Bright was praying for two million to fast and pray for revival before the year 2000, and the Holy Spirit just touched my heart and said, "I want you to do that." I wasn't really scared. I was eager.

One of the major breakthroughs was with our church. I've had nine people who had never fasted before tell me that they want to fast. Four of those people have since fasted and prayed for forty days. Another person has started fasting one day a week. Previously she had told me, "I could never fast for a whole day."

Although we had never talked about fasting in my church before, God used our initial fasting efforts and has really changed that now. It's not that I talk a lot or speak publicly about fasting. But for the last seven years our church has designated March for a prayer emphasis; this year it's going to be *fasting* and prayer.

I believe that whatever issues, whatever sin, whatever problems and circumstances that we want breakthroughs in, He wants us to get to the point of brokenness and a contrite heart. Fasting and prayer is the only thing that can bring me to that level. The closer you draw to God, the more you see your heart. God has shown me that most of the things He reveals to me are for me to *pray.*

I've learned what it means to walk by faith and not by sight. I'm the type who likes to be in control, I like to analyze things and see the end. I'm a counselor therapist, so I like to see results. In the past, I have seen the end and have wanted to take the steps to reach that end. But God has shown me how to take a step without knowing what the end is, and then just wait on Him for the next step. That is a miracle for me to not work toward an end, but to say, "Okay, God." I can now walk by faith and not by sight—God has freed me of needing to be in control. I'm really trusting Him.

It's really the Lord. There's no way I could fast forty days on my own.

⌁

If you are serious enough about the personal and social tasks before you as a Christian to take up the discipline of fasting, you can expect resistance, interference, and opposition. Plan for it, insofar as you are able. Do not be caught unawares. Remember that you are attempting to advance in your spiritual journey and to gain ground for the Kingdom. That necessitates taking ground away from the enemy—and no great movement of the Holy Spirit goes unchallenged by the enemy. I encourage you to find a prayer partner who will stand with you when you fast—to offer intercession for you as you endeavor to seek the Lord through this spiritual discipline.

—Elmer L. Towns
Fasting for Spiritual Breakthrough

Susan

If you have ever wanted to avoid fasting but felt God was leading you in that direction, Susan's testimony will encourage you. She lives in South Carolina.

I entered the fast with a right relationship with God, having confessed all known sin to Him. But during the time of my fast there was an overwhelming sense of my sins. God brought to mind things that I had long since buried from my heart and mind. He showed me areas of pride, jealousy, and a critical spirit. Sadness that my sin hurt Him was a stark reality, perhaps unlike any other time of confession and repentance.

I noticed during the fast a keen sense of His prompting me to pray. One night I was wide awake with a sense of urgency to pray. At 12:45 a.m., I began to pray for a friend in another state. I just followed God's prompting. At 1:15 the phone rang, and it was my friend. She had crawled out of bed at 12:45 and said that if she was still awake at 1:15 she would call me. We talked and prayed for the next hour over the phone.

I awoke one night at 3 a.m. and prayed for one of the people I am discipling. I had no idea what might be going on. I found out the next day that her grandmother had taken ill that morning around the same hour. Incidents like these happened over and over during my fast. Even now I want to continue to listen to His prompting in my heart when He wants me to pray.

I was able to see His faithfulness to me throughout the fast as He sustained me. After about day four or five, I felt better physically than I had ever felt. My energy level was up. I was totally amazed that I could go that long without food.

I remember thinking a year ago, after reading your book, "I don't want to be one of those God calls to fast for forty days." Now I'm so grateful that He did call me.

∾

Stick with me, friends. Keep track of those you see running this same course, headed for this same goal. There are many out there taking other paths, choosing other goals, and trying to get you to go along with them... All they want is easy street. They hate Christ's Cross. But easy street is a dead-end street. Those who live there make their bellies their gods... All they can think of is their appetites. But there's far more to life for us (paraphrase of Philippians 3:17–20).

—Eugene H. Peterson
The Message

Michael

A homemaker, Michael and her family live in California, where they minister to servicemen. She shares how she arranged her schedule to fast even though she has several children at home.

Initially, I wrestled with the concept of fasting all day for forty days. I was relieved to read in *The Coming Revival* of the person who chose to fast only his lunch hour. As a wife and a mother of five, I felt this was more within the realm of possibility for me considering that I would still need to prepare meals for them. I decided to turn my lunch time into a prayer time whenever I could. I wanted to share my experience because I suspect there may be some who will be intimidated by the suggested forty days of fasting. I want them to know that the Lord is faithful to His Word that "if you seek me with your whole heart, you will find me," and "draw near to God and He will draw near to you."

The Lord was so gracious to reveal Himself to me during my devotions. I was overwhelmed by Him! Never before have I been so consistently aware of His presence. I gained a new understanding of His awesome holiness and His unrelenting desire for me to be holy. Never before have I been so conscious of my own sinfulness and self-centeredness. I would spend hours with Him sometimes. Often I found myself weeping with emotion I'd never known. Never before have I had such a deep burden for the need of God's people to repent.

I am so hungry for His presence and His Word and am increasingly able to recall Scripture in my conversations with others. Scripture memorization is no longer something I feel I should do, but something I realize I must do because His Words are "not just idle words for you, they are your *life*" (Deuteronomy 32:47).

Fasting for any extended period can facilitate that wholehearted drawing near to God. He will certainly draw near and be found.

⤳

Jesus went out of his way to embrace the unloved and
unworthy, the folks who matter not at all to the rest of
society—they embarrass us, we wish they'd go away—to
prove that even "nobodies" matter infinitely to God...Jesus
proved in person that God loves people not as a race or
species, but as individuals. We matter to God. "By loving
the unlovable," said Augustine, "You made me lovable."

—Philip Yancey
The Jesus I Never Knew

Tony

*Tony is president of the Riverwoods Christian Center in Illinois, a
facility that provides resident camping opportunities for children
and families from poverty areas near Chicago. His fast began out
of concern for a sick person, then took a different direction. You
will be thrilled to hear what happened.*

In November 1995, I read *The Coming Revival* and began
praying about a twenty-one day fast. God prompted me to
begin at the end of November. The purpose of this fast
was to intercede in prayer for a dying cancer patient. The
Lord then prompted me to shave my head as an outward
sign of my intercession for this cancer patient. I was way
out of my comfort zone, regarding both fasting and the
shaving of my head, but God kept prompting my heart
until I finally conceded and began to fast. Although I was
prompted to fast at a very busy time of year when I needed to be doing year-end fundraising (the board was very
concerned about my shaved head at this time), the Lord's
leading could not have been more clear.

Although fasting was a new experience for me and the
head-shaving made me feel very self-conscious, it ended
up being an incredibly wonderful experience.

By the end of the twenty-one days, the Lord gave me three dreams that were very clear and had powerful interpretations, all of which came true by the end of February. The first dream was that the truth was in "Haz Darr." After much research, I found out that "Haz Darr" is Hebrew for God bringing order to a person's life, or God arranging the life of a person. I felt that He wanted to arrange my steps and that I needed to trust Him completely; He was going to bring about a new thing in my life.

The second dream was related to a demonic deliverance. At a conference, a young woman was delivered from three demons. I had never seen anyone delivered of demons in all the years of my ministry, not to mention being involved in the actual deliverance proceedings.

The third dream was related to my wife and me being called to expand our ministry to healing, deliverance, evangelism, and discipleship. I believe the Lord used fasting to quicken my heart to more clearly hear His leading in these crucial matters of my life.

I invited people to join me in a two-day fast at our camp headquarters in April 1996. The Lord beautifully drew fifteen pastors and lay leaders to join me for the two days. Another ten persons came and went during that time. Most of the participating pastors told me that they had never fasted before in their lives. They all left Riverwoods convinced that they wanted to have a multiple-day annual fast with their congregations.

I believe the Lord has profoundly touched me in new ways through the leading of His Holy Spirit and fasting.

و

One of the greatest ways God changes me is by bringing Scripture to mind I have hidden deep in my heart. And He always picks the right Scripture at the right time. What a reason for staying in His Word daily—reading, studying,

devouring it. And then what a challenge to stay so sensitive
to the Holy Spirit's speaking that He can reach down and
recall just exactly what I need at the very minute I need it.

—Evelyn Christenson
"Lord, Change Me!"

Dennis

*Dennis, who lives in Texas, experienced what many Christians
who commit themselves to doing God's will find—that Satan puts
roadblocks in the way. But God promises that we can defeat
Satan through our Lord Jesus Christ (1 Corinthians 15:57).*

The first day of the forty-day fast, my left eye started doing
very strange things. Doubt set in and I began thinking
about a detached retina, surgery, time away from work—
and abandoning the fast. I began rebuking Satan and
telling him that he would not stop the fast. It only got
worse. I couldn't see to work, so I walked into a room
where I was alone and started praising Jesus whatever the
outcome. The moment I said "Jesus" out loud, it stopped
and never came back.

The fasting was not difficult at all, and it did not interfere with work or household responsibilities. However, it
was a very dry time spiritually. Praying was very difficult
and I didn't hear anything from God. It was like being in
the wilderness.

During a prayer vigil at my church, the Lord impressed
on me that I should share the testimony of my fast with
the congregation. I knew I'd first have to get the senior
minister's permission to do that, and I was very uncomfortable. I asked, "But Lord, what if I didn't get it right?
What if I didn't hear you correctly?" I clearly heard,
"Dance with Me! Whenever you hear Me, dance with Me.
Concerning speaking to this congregation about fasting,
dance with Me."

Four days after completing the forty-day fast, I heard the Lord say, "I will continue to reveal Myself to you if you will continue to pray and fast." I committed to fast at least one day each week.

The following week, the church service started with praise during which people started weeping and kneeling all over the congregation. The pastor abandoned the regular service and had us keep on praising while he read the Bible. After the Scripture reading, he asked me to come up and share. Never had my words flowed so smoothly while I shared Bill Bright's prophecy and my testimony about fasting and "dancing" with the Lord.

The Lord has continued to reveal Himself almost daily through reading the Word and in my journaling. Although the time during the fast was very dry spiritually, since the fast, I have never been closer to the Lord. I continue to stumble, fall, and feel awkward and clumsy, but the Lord is teaching me to "dance" and He will make a beautiful thing of it.

The Lord keeps impressing on me to wait upon Him— especially Psalm 37:8, "Do not fret—it only causes harm" (NKJ); Hebrews 6:15, "After waiting patiently, Abraham received what was promised"; and Psalm 37:34, "Wait for the Lord and keep his way. He will exalt you to inherit the land."

↬

Look carefully then how you walk! Live purposefully and worthily and accurately, not as the unwise and witless, but as wise (sensible, intelligent people), making the very most of the time [buying up each opportunity], because the days are evil. Therefore do not be vague and thoughtless and foolish, but understanding and firmly grasping what the will of the Lord is…Ever be filled and stimulated with the [Holy] Spirit.

—Ephesians 5:15–18 (Amplified)

Gary

Gary, an associate pastor in a North Carolina church, realized how he had lost his first love for the Lord. Because of his fast, he now has a new excitement for serving God.

I am beginning to see just how much materialism and worldliness have us in bondage. Are we really sold out to God like we think we are?

When I was first saved, I experienced the supernatural anointing and presence of God in my daily life. God seemed to direct my path in every way. Something began to happen, and gradually I lost that anointing and close fellowship with the Lord. I have prayed for years for that anointing to return and for the Lord to be real to me again.

When I decided to fast, my wife gave me opposition because of her concern for my health. A staff member called it ridiculous and couldn't understand why I was doing it. Many people kept warning that I was going to ruin my health, and I would tell them, "If God tells us to fast, then it must be good for us."

Dr. Bright, my life is so different now. I began to abide in Him again and He is abiding in me, and as a result I don't have to go out and try to bear fruit; I just automatically do it. I am even surprising myself at the things I am doing. I share Jesus as a way of life again like I used to do. I have such a strong desire to serve my wife and others as well. I have found myself speaking the Word of God with wisdom and boldness. The Word just comes alive as I read it like it did before. I just praise His name for His faithfulness and working in my life.

God allowed me to lead a friend to faith in Jesus as his Savior. I had been praying for him since I was saved in 1973. My brother-in-law for whom I have been praying during my fast was also saved. One couple who was about to separate was convicted by the Holy Spirit and both were saved and joined the church.

One thing is certainly evident—the sanctified life of one person sanctifies another. May the Father help us to be sanctified.

ॐ

God will honor humility. God will honor brokenness. God will honor the fact that we take this time to fast and pray, and God is able to do exceedingly abundant, ... more [than] we could ask or think.

—Dr. Julio Ruibal
Fasting & Prayer '95, Los Angeles

Leslie

Leslie works with students on the campus of West Virginia University. Because of his deepened relationship with Christ, he was able to lead students to a greater faithfulness in their spiritual life.

Because I didn't want this year (1995–96) to be "normal" and "passive" in seeking the Lord, I struggled with how and when I would fast for forty days.

Our first Campus Crusade for Christ outreach came the first day of classes in the fall of '95. It seemed everyone had the same old attitude of being lukewarm. Only fifteen to twenty nonbelievers came out. We had passed out over 2,000 flyers. I asked the Lord, "Why didn't you use us?"

That night the Lord placed deep conviction in my heart. It was as if He said, "Are you ready for me to bring the lost to you? Are you humble and broken to allow My power to draw others to Myself?" That night I knew I needed to seek Him through the forty-day fast. My heart wasn't what God had wanted. I wasn't humbly walking with Him.

About two weeks later, one of our students was hospitalized will a serious illness. She was in critical condition and on a respirator. Our students rallied and prayed in the hospital chapel for her life to be spared. Four months later (three-and-a-half of it on a respirator), Angela was released from the hospital. God had given me the "ability" to lead the students, helping them focus on His love and faithfulness and sovereignty.

> *I asked the Lord, "Why didn't you use us?" It was as if He said, "Are you ready for me to bring the lost to you? Are you humble and broken to allow My power to draw others to Myself?"*

As I look back, more than anything else I am aware that the Lord drew me to Himself. I experienced a deeper intimacy than I have ever known since becoming Spirit-filled. Over and over the Lord sustained me with the juices and broth. I'm more in love with the Lord and more intimate in my relationship with Him than ever before.

༄

If we really believe that God will answer our prayers for revival, then we need to prepare ourselves for the answers before they come. A concert of prayer can be as much an escape from the cause of Christ as attending a rock concert! We can busy ourselves in a cozy group that prays for the world with no real intention of getting further involved.

—David Bryant
Concerts of Prayer

Fred

Fred is senior pastor at a church in Georgia. He describes his forty-day fast as the most wonderful five weeks in his life. He is excited about the answers to prayer he received.

In May, God began to impress on my heart that He would be calling our church to an extended time of prayer and fasting before the fall ministries. The word that God kept speaking to my heart was, "I am working. I want to revive my flock at Lilburn. Go the distance. Don't come up short. Endure to the end."

As different spiritual and moral needs surfaced in our congregation, the Holy Spirit was bringing deeper conviction on my own heart that I needed to fast far longer than three days. The quiet, loving nudging of the Holy Spirit to fast forty days seemed more than challenging; it actually became desirable. In a day of both desperate need and tremendous opportunities, I need to seek God as He desires me to seek Him—with all of my heart.

On October 4, 1995, I completed my forty-day fast. Those five-and-a-half weeks were the most wonderful weeks of my life. There is not even a close second. God's own dear presence has never been so intimate with me and His Word has never been so precious.

After going through the forty-day fast, I can now say that the benefits far exceeded even my wildest dreams. Isn't that just like God?

I am impressed to share that I have logged more than one hundred specific, and in some cases dramatic, answers to prayer, and each day the number is increasing.

↪

Always aim to show kindness and seek to do good to one another and to everybody. Be happy [in your faith] and rejoice and be glad-hearted continually (always); be unceasing in prayer [praying perseveringly]; thank [God] in everything [no matter what the circumstances may be, be thankful and give thanks], for this is the will of God for you [who are] in Christ Jesus [the Revealer and Mediator of that will]. Do not quench (suppress or subdue) the [Holy] Spirit; do not spurn the gifts and utterances of the prophets [do not depreciate prophetic revelations nor despise inspired instruction or exhortation or warning]. But test and prove all things [until you can recognize] what is good; [to that] hold fast.

—1 Thessalonians 5:15–21 (Amplified)

Mark

Mark, who lives in Kentucky, works with a Campus Crusade ministry called Christian Leadership, which reaches out to college faculty. The ministry's main thrust is to bring the Christian worldview back into the campus community in a credible, reasonable manner. They are trying to get Christian faculty to take a stand—to "come out of the closet" for Christ.

I love to eat. Food is one of my favorite things, so I prayed, "God, I'm willing, but I have no will power in this area; I have no strength." Ten years earlier I had tried a one-and-a-half-day fast and barely got through it. I knew God was going to have to do it, but I was willing.

I did see a lot of changes as a result of my fast. My walk with the Lord was the deepest I had ever experienced in twenty years of walking with Him. I began to see victory over private sin that nobody else knew about—a victory that I hadn't seen consistently in my Christian life. That was incredibly liberating and satisfying. As a result, my relationship with my wife became deeper because I began to open up to her about some personal things. Since I wanted to be right with the Lord, I knew that meant I had to be right with people, starting with my wife.

If the Lord can get me through a forty-day fast, He can do it with anybody if they want it seriously. Because of my effort in fasting, several others I know of have begun fasting one day a week or three to five days every so often.

One significant thing happened toward the end of my fast. I was praying that several groups with which we work would be more united in their efforts for a week-long outreach planned for the week before Easter. You may have heard about the revival on Christian campuses that happened in 1996. A part of that revival came to Asbury College—one of the places where we were holding an Easter outreach. Two Wheaton students spoke, and for literally hours into the night people were getting right with the Lord. That happened for three days in a row.

I believe that the revivals we saw a year ago were exciting and tremendous, but I think a critical mass is still to be gathered. I feel that God can begin to work when ordinary people like me get together and do this. At some point—I don't know what the critical mass is—I'm sure it's coming.

I had some spiritual struggles and attacks toward the end of the fast, but not in the way that I expected. I was really caught off-guard. They were physical ailments. I expected attacks or harassment for being a Christian in the campus arena. I wasn't thinking at all about anything physical. I needed some minor surgery and that really discouraged me. I was a little angry at God when it finally began to click, "Hey, this is a spiritual battle going on here." As I recognized what was happening, I began to see victory again.

During the fast, I decided that as a service to my wife and two young boys, I would do the cooking. It actually turned out to be very pleasurable. I was able to serve them a delicious meal, then excuse myself to do some work I needed to do.

One remarkable breakthrough that I saw after the fast was at the University of Lexington. I had been working with a few Christian professors there trying to encourage a greater ministry on campus. After the fast, the ministry seemed to come together in a stronger way—and these three professors began to own it for themselves, rather than my "beating the drum" and doing the recruiting.

૩

I commend to you the reading of biographies of men and women who have been used by God in the church throughout the centuries, especially in revival. And you will find this same holy boldness, this argumentation, this rea- soning, this putting the case to God, pleading His own promises. Oh, that is the whole secret of prayer, I some- times think... Do not leave Him alone. Pester Him, as it were, with His own promises. Tell Him what He has said He is going to do. Quote the Scripture to Him. And, you know, God delights to hear us doing it, as a father likes to see this element in his own child who has obviously been listening to what his father has been saying. It pleases him. The child may be slightly impertinent; it does not matter. The father likes it in spite of that. And God is our Father, and He loves us, and He likes to hear us pleading His own promises, quoting His own words to Him, and saying, "In light of this, can You refrain?" It delights the heart of God.

—David Martin Lloyd-Jones
Revival

Anne

Anne experienced what most of us have during an extended fast: the painful examination of our sin and the grace of God's forgive- ness. Her story will touch your heart.

The forty-day fast with Jesus Christ moved me from being an unstable Christian who constantly battled my own shortcomings, insecurities, and failures to *knowing* that I was God's child in a fresh new way. I felt so completely loved, so cleansed, so able (without striving) to live the

Christian life with a power I had never experienced before, even though I had accepted the Lord as my Savior as a very young child.

I cannot begin to say the ways in which the Lord blessed me by calling me into this fast. Forty days is a very long time to fast—and it seemed that more invitations to parties and food-centered events came up than at any other time. Most of them were easy to pass up. I was happy to be at home centered on the Lord. Never before had I been so moved by Scripture and felt the Holy Spirit teaching me its depth. I'd weep as I read the words that I had so often glossed over before. Often I'd be awakened suddenly in the night with a deep insight as to God's leading or a grasp of spiritual truth.

Time and again the Lord would disclose areas of my life over which I had tried for years to gain victory without lasting results. "You don't trust Me" came to my heart over and over again. I saw how my lack of trust in Him had affected every area of my life—work, relationships, home, and most decisions. After deeply repenting, I now experience tremendous advances in trusting my Lord.

So much of my forty days before the Lord seemed to be "machete" work of clearing a path. I had many glorious moments, but a lot of it was seeing my sin through His eyes. After the fast, I felt God's judgment very strongly for the way I had acted in a past relationship. So many sins came flooding before me; I felt overwhelmed and profoundly sad. That was a hard thing to bear, but also very freeing. I had been carrying around a lot of negativity toward God regarding the past. Finally, I dealt with my responsibility and sin, and this burden slid off me. I also felt led to call that person (after eight years) and ask for forgiveness for my actions. We ended the conversation by forgiving each other.

There were many unique and even funny things that happened as well. For instance, one morning I spent a long time looking for a Scripture reference but could not find it in any of my concordances. I decided to put it off until later and sat down to do my devotions. I flipped the page on a verse-for-the-day calendar. Right there was the Scripture (and reference) I had been searching for! I had to laugh. It was as if God had set this up for me.

While my life is far from perfect, nothing seems to grip me and bring me down like it did before. The presence of the Lord is very real to me all the time, and the Word remains fresh and alive. He is so very good and kind beyond all measure.

∾

Do not be anxious about anything, but in everything,
by prayer and petition, with thanksgiving, present
your requests to God. And the peace of God, which
transcends all understanding, will guard your
hearts and your minds in Christ Jesus.

—Philippians 4:6,7

Daniel

Daniel works with Here's Life New York. When he realized that his walk with the Lord was becoming routine, he began to seek a deeper relationship with God. His fast was part of that change.

One day a friend was talking to me about Jesus and his time with the Lord. His love was so strong for Christ that he started crying over the grace of God. Something in my spirit moved as I realized that I was living a lot of my Christian life "by the numbers." I realized that I wasn't walking with God like my friend was. I wanted it, and that's just what he told me, "You have to want it."

After really seeking the Lord, I had a powerful experience with the Holy Spirit that helped me to sense His presence in a deeper way. It was a personal revival.

I attended the Fasting & Prayer '95 conference in Los Angeles. What started as a three-day fast became extended as the Lord began to lead me to pray for four areas of my life. I spent many hours in prayer simply seeking His direction.

The Lord began to deal with me immediately in a beautiful way. The more I spent time in His presence, the more I was convicted of how feeble my prayer life had been. The Lord showed me that, like Mary, the one thing I needed was to sit at the feet of Jesus. The closer I would draw to God, the more He would reveal Himself to me. I had such a tremendous time with the Lord as He gently led me to understand His will.

> *We want the power of God to be manifested, but sometimes we fail to seek purity on our part.*

My preoccupation with ministry techniques was put aside. The key is the Spirit of God: Is He present or not? He showed me that His will is knowable in specific ways. He showed me that the only way to pray was to seek His will so that I could pray in faith.

I also asked God to show me my sin and to help me overcome certain areas of my life that I knew were not pleasing to Him. He showed me that I had to rise up against these areas, that it was His will for me to be a strong overcomer. He showed me that some of my sins— like a critical spirit, lateness, and anger—were a result of lack of faith. He also showed me my need to simply receive the love of God to overcome my fear of man and fear of loving others. The Lord gave me a vision of a log that first had to be stripped and cleaned before it could be used in the building of a structure. This applied to me directly—I had to be broken in will, mind, and emotion.

The Lord also showed me that we must always stand for purity and power and that nothing should separate these two. Some believers or churches major on power— gifts of the Spirit, anointing, praying with authority, spiritual warfare, healing. And some believers and churches major on purity—purity of doctrine, purity of life, holiness. They need to be brought together and not separated. We want the power of God to be manifested, but sometimes we fail to seek purity on our part.

The Lord also gave me a burden to persevere in prayer, to go boldly before the throne of grace. He impressed upon me that now is the time to pray big prayers, to come into agreement with saints all over the world for this revival. We must see that this is the only way. The Lord has given me a *confident desperation* for Him and for this revival. I really believe that God has this coming revival for us and that it's imminent. He is working to bring our attention to this. I'm also sure that it's not going to happen without the united prayer of the people and going through the process of breaking up the fallow ground with persistent prayer, repentance, obedience— and really seeking it. We need to enter into the burden for it, seek God's face, and, like Jacob, not let go until there's a blessing.

᠅

Upon that cross of Jesus mine eye at times can see
The very dying form of One who suffered there for me;
And from my smitten heart with tears two wonders I confess,
The wonders of his glorious love and my unworthiness.
I take, O cross, thy shadow for my abiding place;
I ask no other sunshine than the sunshine of His face;
Content to let the world go by, to know no gain nor loss,
My sinful self my only shame, my glory all the cross.

—Elizabeth C. Clephane
Beneath the Cross of Jesus

Vicki

Vicki and her husband have been Campus Crusade staff members for seventeen years, currently serving on the campus in Texas.

Her personal revival began at our 1995 staff training. As you read, you will see how her fasting directly impacted her family.

During the 1995 Campus Crusade summer staff training when Nancy Leigh DeMoss spoke on brokenness[2], revival broke out among the staff, and I was really moved.

There were some things going on in our personal life with our daughter and her boyfriend at that time. They had dated for five years, but we had some apprehensions about him because some things had happened. When we were at staff training, our daughter's boyfriend called us and asked my husband if he could marry her. My husband gracefully said yes.

After he got off the phone, I asked my husband what the Lord had said to him to enable him to so very gracefully give his permission for the engagement. He said, "The Lord told me to honor my daughter and to give her the freedom to make her choices." God had to deal with pride in our lives and had to break us to be able to love this young man.

Their wedding was planned for May, but we were still not sure the wedding was going to happen. As it got closer and closer, I prayed that I would be willing to do everything I could do so that His will would definitely be done. I also wanted my heart to be right about their marriage if that was the Lord's will. So I read *The Coming Revival* again in March. On April 7, I felt again strongly that I should do the forty-day fast.

In my time with the Lord, it was like He said, "Vicki, do you think Satan would be telling you to go without food for forty days? It's now or never. Are you going to be obedient and trust Me? Are you willing to pay the price and be sold out?" My heart's desire at that time was that He would be supreme in this wedding and that He would be lifted up and His name exalted. I claimed Romans 2:4 for the wedding, that they would see the Lord's goodness and that it would draw them to Him and to repentance.

On April 9, I said, "Okay, Lord." I fasted for thirty-five days. During that time, there were wedding showers and parties. God was gracious in that no one pressed me about my not eating. My husband kept saying, "I don't think this is a good time to be fasting. Are you sure this is what you should be doing?" If I had gone forty days, it would have been exactly up to the day of the wedding. On that thirty-fifth day, it was just like the Lord said, "This is all. Your heart was right. It's not the logistics of forty days. I just wanted your heart."

One of the things I had prayed for was finances, because as staff members, we didn't want to go into debt. We really wanted to have a beautiful wedding that would honor the Lord, and to have it all paid for. The Lord not only showed His goodness to my daughter and son-in-law, but to us as well. One of the women's Bible study groups that I lead prepared all the food for the wedding as their gift. That was a wonderful answer from the Lord.

We had a '65 Mustang that we had tried to sell, but it hadn't sold. Now it sold in time for the wedding. We were able to pay for the wedding and pay some other debts as well. Not only were we not in debt after the wedding, we didn't owe anything to anyone! It was over and above what we had asked.

I've seen a real healing from the wedding and since that time. My daughter is also growing in the Lord. As parents, we all want godly mates for our children, and we also prayed that our children would love the Lord with all of their hearts, souls, and minds. As we released her and said, "Lord, not what we want," He seemed to say that sometimes He has to do things that are not our ways to ultimately get what we ask for. My husband learned through all this that we didn't really know what love was all about. It cost us giving up and surrendering. It's still not over though. God is working on all of us, and there are still changes that are needed.

I was very happy that *The Coming Revival* mentions that there is nothing wrong with telling other Christians when you're fasting. I had been raised not to tell anyone. God used my testimony to encourage other people.

One of the greatest things about the fast was that my walk with the Lord was closer than at any other time. Also, I had a real sensitivity to the Holy Spirit and hearing and knowing His voice. It's real clear now, where it wasn't previously. Before, I think I was hearing His voice, but it was almost as though I was in a fog. I wasn't being obedient. After going through the fast, I know the voice. I'm also much more aware of when I disobey Him. I want Him to get all the glory.

෴

With his own pangs of hunger, Rees Howells sent up a continual cry to God for the relief of the sufferers whose burden he was carrying...He saw that the point of fasting is to bring the body into subjection to the Spirit. "Each fast, if carried out under the guidance of the Holy Spirit, means that our bodies become more equipped to carry burdens."

—Norman Grubb
Rees Howells, Intercessor

Jewel

Jewel is a businessman from Arkansas. When he began fasting, he did not expect to see God work in his business. His testimony is further evidence that God responds in many different ways to our fasting and prayer.

My wife and I had attended the first Fasting & Prayer gathering in Orlando, and I kept thinking that one of these days I would do a forty-day fast. I had not done more than a three-day fast until that time.

A while after that, we had a crisis in our shopping center business. It was necessary for us to get a new loan on our center, and we had a deadline that we had to meet. The people who held our long-term loan would have liked us to default so they could take over the shopping center. A large mortgage banking firm that was working with us said they would give us the loan, but about forty-five days before the deadline, the vice president of the company called to say they would *not* make the loan. He had just been fired along with 1,500 employees. They were not making *any* loans.

Here we were, right against the deadline, frantically wondering, "What can we do?" One night I awoke at about two o'clock in the morning. I got up and read the Bible awhile and prayed for a considerable period of time, asking the Lord about these various things. After that, it came to my mind again that one of these days I'll do a forty-day fast.

The Lord spoke to me clearly in a strong solid voice, "Why are you waiting?" I was taken aback. I'm used to talking to Him all the time but had never had Him speak to me before. I started weeping. I went in and woke my wife, Eva. Here I am in the middle of the night, crying. She was so startled. When I regained my composure, I said, "I'm starting a fast today because the Lord just spoke to me."

I started that day with juices and had no problem fasting. I didn't even feel hungry. That amazed me because I like to eat! The Lord enabled me to do it.

We went right on with the business, trying to get new leases in our spaces and put together a deal to get a loan. We did get the loan approved before the deadline, so I was able to pay the bank off completely. As I drove away from the bank, the Lord spoke to me for the second time in a very quiet voice, "Your forty days are up tomorrow."

Then it struck me that the fast and the loan had happened at the same time. It didn't occur to me that there was any connection between the two until that moment. I did not fast in order for the Lord to give me the loan. The

Lord put this loan together in *thirty-nine days*. We had been trying months and months to get a loan put together. It came in an unusual way. God just did a miraculous thing for me without my being aware of it at the time.

᪥

His divine power has given us everything we need for life and godliness through our knowledge of him who called us by his own glory and goodness. For this very reason, make every effort to add to your faith goodness; and to goodness, knowledge; and to knowledge, self control; and to self-control, perseverance; and to perseverance, godliness; and to godliness, brotherly kindness; and to brotherly kindness, love. For if you possess these qualities in increasing measure, they will keep you from being ineffective and unproductive in your knowledge of our Lord Jesus Christ.

—2 Peter 1:3,5–8

Linda

Because of the sensitive nature of this story, "Linda" asked that we change her name. Her experiences in fasting are a powerful testimony to God's work in the lives of those who have a heart for Him.

One year ago, I completed a forty-day fast. Along with praying for revival, I felt compelled to pray for freedom from bondage for several people I knew. I saw one friend's life change dramatically, and I know that God continues to work in the others' lives.

One of the people I prayed for was my husband. I had felt a lack of transparency in our marriage, and there were things in my husband's life that caused me to question his intimacy with God. Since I couldn't pinpoint anything, I prayed a lot for him for freedom and truth in the innermost parts. He began to see a counselor on his own initiative,...and as they met, it was made very clear to him that he had an addiction to pornography that began when he was only twelve.

When my husband became a Christian in college, he was aware that pornography was not pleasing to God, and he changed for a while, but it remained a stronghold. Later he shared with me that he had asked God to take it away from him so many times to no avail that he subconsciously concluded that God did not care. He believed that he would have to continue living a mediocre Christian life until God would probably have to end his life to avoid the shame he would bring upon His name. My husband believed that he could never be completely honest with anyone about this issue, especially not with me.

My husband's counselor told him that if he didn't talk to me about this addiction, it would ruin our family. In God's mercy, I happened upon some receipts that my husband had forgotten to dispose of that revealed to me his struggle. When I confronted him, he broke down and told me the truth for the first time. He said that for the first time he felt some hope. Incredibly, I also felt some hope because I finally knew what we were dealing with, and though our hearts were crushed, I knew that God had answered our prayers. The grace of God had prepared me and enabled me to react to my husband in love, which God knew he needed. With tears, my husband said that all he could see was Jesus hanging on a cross telling him over and over that He loved him. My husband realized for the first time that God would not take his life away because of sin, because He already took the life of Jesus.

We both know that God broke chains in my husband's life that day, and that was confirmed as time passed. A few weeks after that fateful day, my husband began a forty-day fast. I think both of us knew that he would not have had the power to do so before.

He continues to talk to me each day and lets me know how he is doing. We have more intimacy in our marriage than I ever expected, and I am so thankful that God is willing to break us in order to answer our prayers and give us the deepest desires of our hearts.

My husband and I are now on the staff of a Christian ministry at a university. Almost every day, my husband is able to share his struggle with young men, which has opened many doors. We've had the privilege of seeing one man open up for the very first time about the same addiction and experience the very same freedom that my husband found from his sin. It is amazing how the Lord uses our worst failures to bring freedom and hope to other people.

> *I am so thankful that God is willing to break us in order to answer our prayers and give us the deepest desires of our hearts.*

After seeing how greatly God worked in our lives personally, we truly believe that He wants to bring revival to others' lives, to our campus, to the nation, and to this world.

⌒

> Create in me a new, clean heart, O God, filled with clean thoughts and right desires. It is a broken spirit you want—remorse and penitence. A broken and a contrite heart, O God, you will not ignore.
>
> —Psalm 51:10,17 (TLB)

Donald

Donald, a Florida state trooper, was looking for direction in his life. The Lord answered through his fast and through prayer.

Currently, I am employed as a state trooper on the Florida Turnpike, but the Lord is leading me out of law enforcement to serve as an evangelist. This fast gave me much-needed direction.

As I began my fast, I encountered an all-out attack from the enemy. My wife reminded me that Satan did not want me to fast and that I needed to pray against the attack and seek the strength and comfort of the Holy Spirit. On day two the attack lifted, releasing me to go on.

I could see that this fast was like a space shuttle breaking free from the gravitational pull of "self" and the "world." I saw myself as one who had heard the plans of our King and left the table to go and do all I could for Him. I now know that I have to go regularly to His table to really know, love, and obey Him. I had preached about having a first love and passion for Christ, but now I was living it.

I felt the presence of the Lord like I never had before. It was like I knew that I was in the presence of an awesome Holy God. At this I heard the Lord say to my heart, "If you will come away for forty days, I will utterly change you." How could I not say yes to such a promise from God?

I then began to notice an incredible sense of unity within my marriage, not just because we were fasting together, but like something broke off us. During the next couple of weeks, the Lord began to free me from other hidden, wrong motivations of my heart. I was freed from the motivation of "man pleasing" and other misleading motives. I saw my wife, as she was led by the Spirit, call her brother at 5:45 a.m. to share with him what the Lord had put on her heart about his backslidden condition. It was like out of the pages of the Bible. She didn't know that he was right in the middle of losing his business to his partner. The timing of her call was perfect, just as he was leaving for the office. This word that she gave to him cut him to the quick, causing him to seriously consider his decision to live for the world. The next week almost half of my wife's family came to our church for the Sunday service. The church is wondering where to find the power we have so that they can be used by God. I have seen for myself that God has His own plan, and fasting and prayer puts me on the same page with Him.

Every day I was experiencing a *sustained* desire and hunger for God...From the apostles to D. L. Moody, from the early church fathers to John and Charles Wesley—all these people who were greatly used of God had something in common. They were all willing to pay the price of losing self in an obedient Spirit-filled life. Many of these also fasted and prayed regularly.

I now feel led of the Lord to a lifestyle of fasting and prayer, to look to the Lord for guidance regarding watching TV and instead spend this time with Him and my family. I also learned to control my appetite when I am eating: to not get second and third helpings; to learn to eat to live, not live to eat; and to stop being mastered by food.

We began to see the Holy Spirit call others to fasting as they saw the fruit in our lives. I would almost start to cry, knowing this was the Lord's work in my heart and His Spirit was speaking through me. I would see the Spirit moving upon a person's heart as He spoke through me.

The Lord placed a strong call in me to evangelize the college campus. He just seemed to clear all the smoke about where I am supposed to go. My wife and I are looking so forward to being sent forth into the ministry to which He called us.

～

We do not lose heart. Though outwardly we are wasting away, yet inwardly we are being renewed day by day. For our light and momentary troubles are achieving for us an eternal glory that far outweighs them all. So we fix our eyes not on what is seen, but on what is unseen. For what is seen is temporary, but what is unseen is eternal.

—2 Corinthians 4:16–18

Kimberly

Kimberly, who lives in Kentucky, tells how she fasted for a family member. Although she did not see immediate answers to her prayers, God was working. Her dramatic account of answered prayer will thrill you.

I'm the youngest of four children. My oldest sister, with whom I have always been very close, has fought an alcohol problem for years. She is divorced with two children. We were raised in a Christian home, and she professed Christ as a young person.

About a year ago, the alcohol problem had really caused some conflict in the stability of her home and with her children. At that time, the Lord was placing it on my heart to fast for her. God impressed upon me that if you want something to the degree that you're willing to sacrifice for it, you will lay your life down for it. The Lord impressed on me that if I wanted my sister to be free, it would take a sacrificial act of fasting.

After some preparation, both mentally and physically, I began fasting. Isaiah 58 kept coming to my mind—to break the bondage and break the yokes. This was a long-standing, ingrained problem. My sister had been involved in the New Age movement in the past, but had come out of that.

After I finished the fast, I didn't see any results, but I knew that was what the Lord wanted me to do. About six months later, my sister moved back to Kentucky. She had been experiencing some horrendous, tormenting dreams of impending doom. It got to the point where she couldn't even sleep or rest. She asked me what she should do. I told her that I thought she needed a deliverance. She finally agreed. In the past, I really couldn't have brought the subject up with her.

I called a few friends who had also prayed for her from time to time to prepare in prayer for a deliverance for her.

We met at my church in one of the rooms with a select group of people, including my pastor, my sister, and myself. That night we began to pray. After about two hours, she was delivered of several demons. We took authority and professed the blood over her life. Her body went rigid, and there was a low growl at times. We sensed that several demons let go and fled. I could feel the vibration in her body. She told us she could hear one laughing in her and that the demon was hiding. I looked into her eyes and said, "You're exposed. By the authority of Jesus Christ you will flee." Finally, the release came.

Later at my home, my sister told me that the demons were talking within her, and that one said as he was leaving, "This kind only comes out through much prayer and fasting."

That was a blessing to me because I knew God can make the demons confess that it was the prayer and fasting that had done that. This has also had an impact on my family and the way they approach my sister's problems. Fasting coupled with prayer can break bondages and barriers that prayer alone won't. It's incredible. It has also increased our faith that deliverance can come.

⁓

The saints and friends of Christ served our Lord in hunger and thirst, in cold and nakedness, in toil and weariness, in watching and fasting, in prayer and meditation, in persecutions and insults without number...Grounded in true humility, they lived in simple obedience, they walked in charity and patience, and thus daily increased in the Spirit, and received great grace from God...Oh, the carelessness and coldness of this present time! Sloth and lukewarmness make life wearisome for us, and we soon lose our early fervour!

Thomas à Kempis
The Imitation of Christ

Daniel

One of the joys of reading these testimonies is seeing how God is using The Coming Revival *in people's lives. Daniel, a salesman from Tennessee, saw God work in his personal life and business.*

In November 1994, I was impressed by the Holy Spirit to begin to know what it was like to deny self, pick up my cross, and follow Him. I felt that God the Holy Spirit was speaking to me, and the way that I would experience denying self would be a prolonged fast. I previously had fasted only for short periods of time.

Soon after that initial impression, I starting reading *The Coming Revival.* I didn't even know it was about fasting. It was really a manual for me and a confirmation to begin a fast.

My wife has multiple sclerosis, and during the fast I frequently prepared meals for her without experiencing any hunger. I saw myself serving her in a way that I've never served her before, really ministering to her, and the Holy Spirit ministering to her through me.

Just a few days before I was to end my fast, I attended a Saturday night service at Pastor Don's church. During the worship time, the enemy attacked me with such strong words of fear and accusations that I was almost hyperventilating. The service was at the point of serving the Lord's Supper. I was glad it was time to get up because I was fidgety. I went down to receive the elements, and as I was standing there two brothers came up to me. (I had not seen them before nor since.) They asked me, "Would you like to share the Lord's body with us?" I said, "Certainly," and then I confessed to them, "I am on a fast, and I am being attacked and need you to pray for me." Just like that, they did. Without asking any questions, they began to pray. As they prayed, I could physically feel all the fear and trembling that had been laid on me lifting from my body. There's no question about it. I was relieved. I went back to my seat and continued in the worship service.

Isaiah 58 tells us of the blessings that come from heart-felt fasting. I'm a salesman, and my business flourished. I've never seen anything like the way it took off. It was just incredible. I really felt the Lord was blessing me. (In this world so full of materialism, I hesitate to talk about a material increase as a definite sign from God.)

Since my forty-day fast, I've been doing a lot more one-on-one counseling with men who are struggling—who know the Lord and are really struggling in it or who haven't really met Him yet.

I am a person who has a particularly addictive personality. For example, I'm not one who knows what it is to eat *one* potato chip. Before I was a Christian, I drank alcohol and didn't know what it was like to drink in moderation. At that time, I was also running with a wealthy crowd and eating lots of heavy food and meat. The drinking ended in 1977. So nineteen years later, here I am going for forty days without any heavy food. I saw clearly in my fast that heavy eating does feed on itself.

The Lord is faithful in all these things. He commands us to fast, and He equips us to do it. I know it wasn't anything that I would naturally do. He demonstrates clearly His promise, "I can do all things through Christ who strengthens me" (Philippians 4:13).

⌇

Just as worship begins in holy expectancy, it ends in holy obedience. If worship does not propel us into greater obedience, it has not been worship. To stand before the Holy One of eternity is to change...In worship an increased power steals into the heart sanctuary, an increased compassion grows in the soul. To worship is to change.

—Richard J. Foster
Celebration of Discipline

Dal

Dal is president and chairman of Fellowship of Christian Athletes, and lives in Missouri. As you might guess, he has a deep love for sports and ministry. His testimony emphasizes the importance of humility.

I've always been somewhat of an overachiever. I felt like I could outwork everybody. I'm a football player and a football coach by profession and worked for thirty-nine years in organized football. Being a guy of small stature, I had to hustle to outwork and outperform so I could achieve the various goals I had set for myself. I was very much goal-oriented and a workaholic type over the years. One of the things that I've experienced is a personality change. Not necessarily just because of the forty-day fast, but I've been seeking to do some refining as a result, trying to bring some rhythm and balance into my life.

> *I don't think you can have an intimate relationship with your wife until you have an intimate relationship with the Lord.*

Basically, football was just about my god for a long time. The Lord used the Fellowship of Christian Athletes to help me understand that. The Lord has really revealed personality traits so that my sensitivity is much stronger. I still have the tendency to think that sixteen-hour work days are just average. Even though I had talked about putting the Lord first and my wife and children next and putting football back where it belonged, I was not doing that with FCA.

Ministry—being in the people business—can be a 24-hour, 365-day job. Consequently, if I'm not careful, I can let ministry dominate everything. I really had to take the time to look inside again and say, "Lord, help me to distinguish between my goals and your goals."

Also, my wife and I have been married nearly forty years. I don't think you can have an intimate relationship with your wife until you have an intimate relationship with the Lord. Fasting together has really given us a lot more intimacy in our marriage.

I spoke a bit about fasting at a church not long ago, and afterwards the pastor and I continued to talk about it. He said that in forty years he had never fasted or even preached on fasting. He felt the Lord was really speaking to him about that. While we were speaking, one of his deacons joined our conversation. I answered some questions he had about fasting, then he said, "My wife and I have been praying for three months about whether the Lord would have us fast. This just really confirms that this is what we are supposed to do." He made a covenant with the pastor that they would fast and pray together.

When we earnestly put into action that we really do want to deny ourselves and take up our cross and follow Christ in whatever our profession—but especially if we are called to ministry—we need to look inside ourselves and look up to the Father who created us in His image. We need to humble ourselves, pray and seek His face, and repent of our sins. Until we do that, we won't see the church be all that it can be, we won't see families or school campuses being all they should be. This experience of fasting and prayer has really brought into focus how very much we need to be centered on Christ.

◌ᔓ◌

It appears to me that believers generally have expected far too little present fruit from their labors among children.
They hope that the Lord will some day confirm their instruction and answer the prayers which they offer up on the children's behalf... We have to guard against thinking that it does not matter whether we see present fruit or not. On the contrary, we should give the Lord no rest until

we see fruit. Therefore, in persevering yet submissive prayer, we should make our requests known to God.

—George Muller
The Autobiography of George Muller

Darlene

Darlene shares how God is using children in the fasting and prayer movement. She also saw the movement reach into her church. Darlene completed a forty-day juice fast followed by a forty-day "Daniel" fast.

God very clearly called me to be an intercessor. I also have a tremendous heart for the children in my neighborhood. Children are very much a part of this fasting and prayer movement. The Book of Joel says to gather together in solemn assembly the children and the nursing infants. I was glad to see several children and infants at the St. Louis gathering. I see God raising up child prayer warriors that are so mighty that their prayers will astound you.

During my fast, the Lord revealed to me that we are called to trials and affliction. After compiling all the Scripture on affliction, I purposefully set my mind to glorify God in whatever cross He gave me—and that has been absolutely incredible. Right now, we're going through three of the biggest problems that have ever hit us, but the joy and peace that I have are overwhelming. My husband has cancer, he's losing his job, and my daughter is more ill than she's ever been in her life. We see attacks from the Enemy everywhere, yet I can see God moving in such a mighty way through it. He gives me the assurances.

When you fast and pray long-term, set your face like flint, and follow your Savior and carry His cross, every day is a miracle. There's victory after attack, victory after attack—it just goes on all day. God has enabled me to stay awake, and the night watches are absolutely precious. Those are the times I really hear His voice the clearest.

During my forty-day fast, my pastor, who has been instrumental in bringing the prayer movement strongly to our church, was diagnosed with pancreatic cancer and told he had four months to live. The church went into shock. We began to do spiritual warfare through prayer.

That was one of the bigger tests the Lord gave me in this fast. He asked me one day, as I was driving down the freeway, to go to the hospital to lay hands on the pastor and pray for his healing. I said, "Lord, I don't lay hands on pastors and pray for healing. I don't have the gift of healing." When I argue with Him, it just shows how much my flesh is alive. So anyway, He arranged it. Through the prayers of the children and the church, the pastor was completely healed of all cancer. One of the first places the pastor went after he came out of the hospital was to the children's classroom to thank them for their prayers.

At the time of the fast, God warned me, "You want to climb this mountain and go this way, but, my child, count the cost." He gave me three things that I knew very little about: great rejection, great grief, and great loneliness. I didn't want to hear that. He asked, "Would you follow me there? There will be a valley on the other side." I knew I could only say yes to Jesus. What's the alternative?

Henry Blackaby said to a group of intercessors, "You wish to follow the Savior and be the intercessors, but are you really willing to follow Him?" He referred to Isaiah 53 and took it apart line by line. "Are you willing to be 'a man of sorrows, despised and rejected,' etc.?" It absolutely terrified me. "Do you really want to be my son and bear the sorrows of others?" It took me a long time to say yes to those things. But as I have said yes to that, He has allowed just tiny touches of it to come.

On the forty-third day of this fast, the Lord began to show me my sin like never before. I was on my face all day, crying, weeping, and moaning. Later that day, my son sat and wept with me and never said a word. Soon after, I found out that he had been praying strongly all during my fast that God would humble me, because he saw sins in me. You know, your closest loved ones see. He saw the sin of pride and that it needed to be dealt with. People tend to elevate you when they learn you've fasted for forty days—put you on a pedestal. The Lord showed me that I needed to fast for my sin and what was in my heart. It's important not to become arrogant about fasting.

꒰ꋖ

Fasting is a powerful auxiliary weapon, appointed by God, to break the enemy's hold...Satan is a stubborn foe, and will not relinquish his grasp on the spirits and souls, minds and bodies of men unless compelled to do so. Fasting seems to provide that compelling.

—Arthur Wallis
God's Chosen Fast

Becky

Becky is an author and speaker who lives in California. Through her fast, she saw answers to prayer in both her career and her family.

During my partial fast, I saw many answers to prayer. A person close to me who had been unemployed and searching for a job for more than a year received a job offer that was perfectly suited to his gifts and talents. A long-standing dream to tape and produce a daily 90-second radio show, called "Let Prayer Change Your Life," became a reality and ran for twelve weeks prior to the National Day of Prayer. (I had been praying about both of these items daily for more than a year, but the breakthrough seemed to come during the fast!)

I also saw a significant turn of interest in my sixteen-year-old son. Without going into personal details, I believe that the fast expedited a breakthrough in areas that my teenager was struggling with, bringing resolve, peace, clarity, and strength to his daily walk with God!

I knew (and have since proven to myself) that the will power I had to stay on this fast was supernaturally given to me. The general benefits of the fast included: 1) more focus during my daily hour of prayer; 2) an acute awareness that praying and fasting for my sixteen-year-old son during those forty days was more significant than I will ever know; 3) a God-given confidence that I can be a self-controlled, Spirit-controlled Christian woman and leader with the power to abstain when called upon or convicted; and 4) a more conservative taste (and by most standards, I am already very particular) in what I choose to read or watch on TV or at the movies!

It was an *exhilarating* journey. Dr. Bright, without your challenge and example, I would have missed one of the most significant events of my spiritual walk!

⌇

The proper good of a creature is to surrender itself to its Creator...In the world as we now know it, the problem is how to recover this self-surrender. We are not merely imperfect creatures who must be improved: we are, as Newman said, rebels who must lay down our arms...To surrender a self-will inflamed and swollen with years of usurpation is a kind of death...Hence the necessity to die daily: however often we think we have broken the rebellious self, we shall still find it alive.

—C. S. Lewis
The Problem of Pain

Gayle Anne

Gayle Anne worked in my office at the time she underwent this fast. Some time after this experience, the Lord led her into full-time Christian ministry.

During the forty-day fast, I focused on a greater level of worship and intimacy with Jesus and the work of His Spirit in all the earth around me. I felt cleansed, loved, and empowered in the supernatural strength of God. I learned very quickly that I have been very unappreciative of His holiness.

One of the blessings that I will get to testify about for many years to come is the birth of my first nephew, Alexander Robert. My sister and brother-in-law had been trying for several years to have a child. Before entering my fast, I told her that I would faithfully ask God to give her a child soon. Three weeks into my fast, my sister conceived. I know that this will be a vehicle in God's timing to draw their hearts to Him in a personal relationship that they do not now have.

> *I truly came to realize that He delights in blessing those who diligently seek Him.*

I am constantly overwhelmed with God's concern and delight in answering the petitions of His children so creatively and willingly. I truly came to realize that He delights in blessing those who diligently seek Him. My prayer life and vision for His work have changed.

Financial miracles flourished during this fast as well. I prayed to sell a small business I had started and to pay off my business loan. God supernaturally brought someone desiring to start a similar gift business, and she wanted *all* of my inventory. My loan was paid off the same day!

Following the Los Angeles Fasting & Prayer '95 while on standby for a flight, I was the one person selected to get the only seat available on the last plane out. My seatmate for the next five hours was a young, tormented gal wearing black lipstick, black eye shadow, black spiked hair, black clothing, black nails, and a very dark spirit.

After a half hour of just showing her that I cared about who she was, the ground of her spirit was softened to let her in on eternity. Her resistance faded quickly, confirming the Holy Spirit's plan. She was so thirsty for love and acceptance. We flipped from Scripture to Scripture, and I answered her questions. The occult and the New Age movement had been her greatest teachers. Eastern religions clouded her understanding, and she was confused and continually searching, but she was ready and willing to learn something of this thing called "Christianity." I continue to pray for Elizabeth and believe that she will be with me in eternity as the Lord uses this seed in her life.

ᔓ

> Though the doors were locked, Jesus came and stood among them and said, "Peace be with you!" Then he said to Thomas, "Put your finger here; see my hands. Reach out your hand and put it into my side. Stop doubting and believe." Thomas said to him, "My Lord and my God!" Then Jesus told him, "Because you have seen me, you have believed; blessed are those who have not seen and yet have believed."
>
> John 20:26–29

Ralph

Ralph is a dentist whose practice is in Indiana. He is part of an active outreach ministry in his city and participated in a forty-day fast.

My forty-day fast was without a doubt the most significant event in my thirty-year walk with the Lord. I felt great— better, in fact. I did not miss food after the third day, and it was hard to convince people around me that I was not going to hurt myself by not eating.

Aside from all this, my spiritual life soared. It seems that the farther I progressed into the forty-day fast, the closer God was to me. My mind was clearer and difficult decisions were made with unwavering confidence that God was giving me wisdom. I slept better and sounder than usual, and I would awaken with a smile on my face. The usual morning body stiffness was gone, and the Lord and I would start another adventure together.

During this forty-day fast, I did not have to look for a "time" to pray. If I was awake, I was in prayer all the time. He became stronger as I became weaker.

$$\approx$$

Fasting reveals the things that control us. We cover up what is inside us with food and other good things, but in fasting these things come to the surface...It is certainly not a bad thing to feel good, but we must be able to bring that feeling to an easy place where it does not control us. So many attitudes strive to control us: anger, pride, fear, hostility, gluttony, avarice. All of these and more will surface as we fast. It is a blessed release to have these things out in the open so that they can be defeated, and we can live with a single eye toward God.

—Richard J. Foster
Freedom of Simplicity

Dale

Dale is pastor of a church situated on the Mexico/Texas border. How God led him to fast will thrill your heart.

I was at the Promise Keepers meeting for pastors in Atlanta, and I felt this nudge to go on a forty-day fast. At that time, I had never heard of anyone doing a forty-day fast. I thought, "That's crazy, nobody does that." I kept pushing the thought away. I'm a very reluctant faster. Also, I wasn't into heroics or trying to prove anything, so forty days seemed outrageous. Part of me did not believe it was from God.

I was reluctant and asked God if He would confirm it to me. The day before, I had purchased several books, and one was *The Coming Revival*. That next night, I just opened the book and happened to read the part about two million people fasting for forty days. Just like that, I knew that was what I was supposed to do. Still, I didn't really know *why* I was doing it. I didn't have any agenda.

I don't have a "success" story, but I hope you'll feel that it's important to let people know that not everyone does. I wondered if I was doing something wrong. In fact, I started getting migraines; I had itching all over; I got boils on my face a couple weeks after I started. I didn't know if it was a sign that I should stop. I wasn't experiencing any hunger, but other than that I was physically overwhelmed.

I came home from Promise Keepers with a boldness in preaching that I hadn't had before. I had just come as pastor to my church two months earlier. We are situated on the border of Mexico, and the church was not doing well. At that time, there were only thirty-five people attending. There wasn't a lot of hope in the church. I told the congregation that I had begun a forty-day fast, and many of the people supported me. Several decided to fast a day with me or skip a meal. My wife, who was expecting our third child at the time, knew she couldn't fast by going without food, but she fasted other things. That really encouraged and empowered me.

Still, not much happened and I continued to wonder if I was blocking God somehow. So much of what you hear are these wonderful testimonies of changed lives and whole cities changing, etc. I didn't understand, but at least I had the theological training to be able to figure out that God is God. When we fast, we expect something to happen, but God is sovereign even there. He wanted me to fast for His own reason, and I may not know what that is in my lifetime. My part was obedience. It may be that God was dealing with things in my congregation or my life that I know nothing about. I have to trust Him.

In fact, prior to the fast, I felt like my congregation was with me in making some changes. Then they just seemed to go back to where they had been before. One of the things I did get was a still small voice saying that I need to keep my eyes open regarding struggles in the ministry, especially pride. I didn't feel that pride was a problem area, but I listened and watched myself more carefully.

I want to encourage other people who fast and don't see a lot of results. It doesn't mean God is not with you. It doesn't mean you've done something wrong. I don't think we should shy away from mentioning that in a book. Others need to know they are not alone. Perhaps if I had seen big changes in my congregation I would have directly attributed it to *my fast* rather than to God's sovereignty.

> *I want to encourage others who fast and don't see a lot of results. Perhaps if I had seen big changes I would have directly attributed it to* my fast *rather than to God's sovereignty.*

Mother Teresa said, "We are not called to be successful, we are called to be faithful."

Jesus calls us to fast, not because it will make us spiritual giants, but to humble ourselves. There needs to be a balanced witness of what fasting is about. If miracles come, praise Him. If not, there is no condemnation and God loves us. He doesn't jump through our hoops. It's not about us (we can be so self-absorbed)—it's about God.

ॐ

Make a careful exploration of who you are and the work you have been given, and then sink yourself into that. Don't be impressed with yourself. Don't compare yourself with others. Each of you must take responsibility for doing the creative best you can with your own life...Don't be misled: No one makes a fool of God. What a person plants, he will harvest. The person who plants selfishness,

ignoring the needs of others—ignoring God!—harvests a
crop of weeds. All he'll have to show for his life is weeds!
But the one who plants in response to God, letting God's
Spirit do the growth work in him, harvests a crop of real,
eternal life. So let's not allow ourselves to get fatigued
doing good. At the right time we will harvest a good crop
if we don't give up, or quit. Right now, therefore, every
time we get the chance, let us work for the benefit of all,
starting with the people closest to us in the community
of faith (paraphrase of Galatians 6:3–10).

—Eugene H. Peterson
The Message

Daiquin

Daiquin tells how fasting is a powerful weapon that refreshes him spiritually. His testimony comes from Texas.

Every need that I prayed for has been answered. One
prayer was for my wife's diagnosed pre-cancer in the
womb to be healed so we could return wholeheartedly to
China to serve God. During her checkup a week after my
prayer, no cancer was found. I view this as a miracle that
God had given me in mercy and to show that He is still
sovereignly in control. We also saw God answer our
prayers for the restoration of a friend's marriage. The husband has accepted the Lord. Also, a Christian friend was
healed from a kidney disease.

Fasting and prayer is a very powerful spiritual weapon
that has been neglected by the church for a long while. At
this end of an age, all servants of God should learn to take
back this weapon that our Lord Jesus has shown us how to
use. I don't feel it's a matter of showing personal spiritual-
ity, but of total inability and complete dependence on
God our Father. When I feel spiritually low, fasting with
prayer seems to refresh me and put me back on track. I
plan to make it a regular habit of my life and ministry.

✌

The Lord first makes us conscious of our weakness, so that
our heart cries out, "I can't handle this." We go to the
Lord, telling Him, "I can't handle this. Please take it away!"
And the Lord replies, "In My strength you can handle it."
Thus in the end your testimony, like Paul's, will be,
"I can do all things through Christ who strengthens
me" (Philippians 4:13). That, I believe, is the fullest
expression of the empowered Christian life.

—J. I. Packer
"Power for a Purpose," *Discipleship Journal*

Marjorie

*Marjorie's testimony comes from Colorado. Although the portion
we have included is brief, it is a blessing to read.*

I completed a forty-day juice fast with many precious blessings, including the miraculous salvation of a seventy-six-
year-old hardened atheist on the fortieth day. Praise to the
Lord!

✌

As we become single-minded through fasting and prayer,
our spiritual vision comes into focus. Often the Holy Spirit
tries to call us to Himself, but we are slaves to our flesh.
Our faith should not rest in the wisdom of men, but in
the power of the Spirit. We want instant spiritual insight,
but the Lord wants our faithfulness. Faith is militantly
"holding on to that which looks impossible."

—Alice Smith
Power Praying

Churchwide Fasting and Prayer

O ur churches are under attack on several fronts. Many congregations are reeling from the effects of internal and external criticism, the breakup of families, a lack of leadership, financial pressures, and numerous other problems. But God is at work in our churches, bringing us to His desires for ministry and healing. Reading these testimonies of how fasting and prayer have helped revitalize church ministry has filled my heart with praise for God's work in His Church.

As you discovered in "Individual Fasting and Prayer," many churches have been changed for the better through the enthusiasm of individuals who shared their commitment to fasting and prayer. In this section, you will read testimonies of what happens when church members set aside time for fasting and prayer. In each case, one or more Christians felt led of the Lord to fast, then shared their experiences with others in their church. In some instances, the churchwide fasting spread to other churches in the area.

Whether the fast began with just a few people in a congregation or the entire church body, God did marvelous things. Perhaps these examples will inspire you to share your fasting and prayer experiences with the leaders in your church.

If you would like more information about organizing a churchwide fast, my staff and I have prepared a small book called *Preparing for the Coming Revival: How to Lead a Successful Fasting & Prayer Gathering*. It can help you prepare the leadership of your church, establish a movement of fasting and prayer in your church, and conduct a fasting and prayer gathering. Also available is a 25-page reference guide, *Seven Basic Steps to Successful Fasting & Prayer,* that you can share with others to help them begin a fast. (See the Resources section at the back of this book for ordering information.)

Life Center Ministries International

Pastor Charles Stock, from Camp Hill, Pennsylvania, had come to a point in his ministry where he was wondering if the Lord had a new assignment for him. As he tried to determine God's will, the question came back from the Lord, "Why haven't you fasted?" His response affected his entire church and its ministry.

I didn't want to fast. However, with a loving persistency that characterizes the blessed Holy Spirit, the conviction wouldn't go away. If I wanted breakthrough, then my Father was calling me to fast. Not only fast, but fast for forty days. That figure had grown in my heart over the months of wrestling with God on this subject.

I did not feel that it was time to call for a churchwide fast, but did feel I needed to inform the congregation concerning my plans. I wanted as much prayer support as I could possibly get. A week before the fast began, I preached a motivational sermon on fasting. I also invited any who might sense the leading of God to participate for whatever length of time and to whatever degree to do so.

I was not prepared for what happened. There was an overwhelming release of God's grace to me and to the whole congregation for fasting. Children fasted. Teenage boys fasted. All this was voluntary, with no request for a churchwide fast. Easily eighty percent of the congregation fasted in some way for some length of time.

As surprised as I was by the level of participation, I was even more surprised by the manifestations of God's favor that began to occur almost immediately. From the first week, some people began to receive supernatural financial breakthroughs. Houses sold. Fine art sold. Money was given to people who had secret needs. New opportunities opened up for businesses.

The wife of one of our elders conceived and is pregnant after more than twelve years of trying. Physical healings occurred that hadn't been prayed for specifically. A woman was spontaneously healed of inoperable peptic ulcers.

Unbelieving relatives were saved. Estranged parents and children reconciled. Whole houscholds were reunited through a combination of salvations, deliverances, and reconciliations. A family involved in an unjust legal battle not only won the case, but discovered that an anonymous donor had paid the legal fees.

> *As surprised as I was by the level of participation, I was even more surprised by the manifestations of God's favor that began to occur almost immediately.*

It was as if we moved into a whole new era of favor. Many of these painful situations had gone on for years. Ministry ideas were birthed. A couple who had fasted from television received a clear vision and an initial networking to establish a media and communication ministry to serve the Body of Christ.

The other amazing grace story is in how the reputation and favor of the church changed. The church had been plagued with criticism and a kind of under-the-surface instability. We began seeing and hearing from people who attributed all kinds of good things to us, things we didn't deserve or do. Teary-eyed members of the congregation would stop me and thank me for fasting for them. Pastors in the city would give thanks publicly for me and for the congregation for fasting and praying for revival in the city.

During the last twelve days of the fast, the elders met every morning at 5:30 a.m. to pray for breakthrough. These were special times of conviction of sin, confession, repentance, and rejoicing in the tender mercies of God.

Six weeks have passed since the fast ended. There is a different atmosphere in the church. Ministry is opening up all over the region and the world for people from the church. The pastors in the city continue to work and pray for unity. We believe revival is coming. I am looking forward to the next fast that the Lord chooses!

ॐ

When our church has a day of fasting in grief for the sins of our country, we also include prayers asking the Lord to protect and deliver us from enemies that might result from our sins. We realize that He often disciplined Israel for her sins by allowing national enemies to gain advantage over her militarily or economically. Perhaps we don't think as often of the reality of national sin as we should, and how Christians will experience part of any national judgment that comes, even though we did not contribute directly to the national sin.

—Donald S. Whitney
Spiritual Disciplines for the Christian Life

Southwest Church of the Nazarene

Alton R. Hansom is Senior Pastor at the Southwest Church of the Nazarene in Medford, Oregon. What a thrill to read how churches cooperated in teaching about fasting and prayer! Praise God that this is happening in many places.

During a multi-church event in Medford during January 1996, Mr. Chan Keith taught on fasting and prayer. The teaching resulted in a forty-day fast by three churches in Medford. It would seem that God is saying to the Church to repent and humble herself, to learn discipline through fasting and praying, to be in intercessory prayer for the lost. We should all take part in fasting and praying that God would have mercy on us, our country, and the souls of six billion people on our planet.

ॐ

Again, I tell you that if two of you on earth agree about anything you ask for, it will be done for you by my Father in heaven. For where two or three come together in my name, there am I with them.

—Matthew 18:19,20

Manhattan Bible Church

We received two testimonies from the Manhattan Bible Church in New York, illustrating how laymen can help change their church through prayer and fasting. Both accounts show the work of God within a congregation that surrenders itself to His leading.

Roy

Roy is an elder at Manhattan Bible Church and director of New York Gospel Outreach (NY GO), which trains teens from all over the nation to share their faith among the 180 different people groups in New York City.

The members of Manhattan Bible Church readily admit that their church was floundering a couple of years ago. There was a divisive and complaining spirit. Even though great things had happened in the past, there seemed to be a major blockage. Then Roy caught the vision of fasting and prayer for his church, igniting a fire there and beginning a miraculous change.

Roy also initiated a monthly fast day for the church. Several other members in the church have also completed a forty-day fast.

In October 1995, I began to sense a great need for God to bring His power and presence into the life of our church in a greater way. I had previously heard testimony of what

God had done in Dr. Bright's life through a forty-day fast. I felt that through fasting and prayer, in brokenness, we needed Him to bring revival and victory into our lives and into His church. I believed that God was calling me to fast and pray for forty days.

Although not the pastor of our church, I was given the opportunity to speak one Sunday morning. In the eighteen years that God has allowed me to preach and teach His Word, I have never experienced Him speak as powerfully through me as it seemed He did that day. I challenged our congregation to take at least one day to set aside everything and do nothing but pray, fast, and seek the Lord for revival in their lives and in our church. One other man fasted for forty days and another for twenty days. Others began (or continued) fasting on a weekly basis, and many took a day to seek the Lord in prayer and fasting. The elders and their wives began to regularly set aside days to pray and fast together.

Several weeks ago, in our most recent time of prayer and fasting together, there was a spirit of great encouragement over what God has so graciously begun in His church. Over the past several months, members have commented how they now look forward to Wednesday evening services to be inspired by hearing what God has been doing in the lives of our members. It is rare to find a Wednesday service in which the testimony time doesn't end with several enthusiastic members still waving their hands in hopes of testifying of the specific and exciting ways in which they have seen God work.

About four months ago, our pastor shared with the elders that he believed God was leading him to focus more on evangelism and on a traveling and speaking ministry. Although he would remain the founding pastor and a member of Manhattan Bible Church, we would probably need another pastor to focus exclusively on the needs of the local congregation. For six weeks he and the elders met together to pray, fast, and seek the Lord. We unani-

mously agreed that this was the direction God was leading
our pastor and our church. Again, we prayed and fasted as
we anticipated a Sunday evening in which the pastor and
his wife would share with the congregation how they and
the elders believed God was directing.

At this time many members of our congregation were
doing a study called *Experiencing God.* Sovereignly, a large
majority of them had just completed a chapter that dealt
with how a church should
respond to the changes that
God brings. Because our
church had had the same
pastor for over twenty years,
we knew there would be
great room for fear, insecu-
rity, and confusion. Instead,
the result was a time of love
and unity. We provided
another Sunday evening for
the congregation to share
from their hearts, after having had the opportunity to

> *I still found myself
> struggling with...
> sins just as I did
> when I was not fast-
> ing. I had not been
> transformed into a
> "super saint" just
> because my stomach
> was growling.*

pray about this for a month. Again, what the enemy would
have liked to use to bring division and strife in our
church, God used to bring an affirmation of commitment
as we move ahead into the work God has for us.

One thing that was interesting about my forty-day fast
was that I still found myself struggling with pride, selfishness, anger, and other sins just as I did when I was not fasting. I had not been transformed into a "super saint" just
because my stomach was growling. What I did find was
that I seemed more spiritually alert and sensitive to God
than I ever was before.

In addition to all I learned during my fast, I believe
that God laid the foundation for some deeply significant
things He would teach me after my fast was completed. I
believe God has been teaching me in an ongoing way how

to listen more carefully and specifically as He speaks to me. He has also been teaching me how to obediently apply what He says to me each day. God began a work in my life and in our church that I do not believe I would have been a part of had I not been obedient to seek the Lord in prayer and fasting.

ଏ

Humility is at the heart of fasting. Humility is a quality that manifests itself in how one acts in relation to God and others. It is to lower one's estimate of self by elevating one's estimate of others. And because fasting carries this quality of humility into the tangible, physical realm, it brings about a brokenness before God that can come in no other way. Such brokenness not only honors God but makes the intercessor's heart more pliable to hear from Him. He is thus more useful in carrying out God's Kingdom plans.

—Dick Eastman
Love On Its Knees

Tony

Tony is a New York City policemen who continued his stressful job while completing a forty-day fast. He admits to previously being unable to fast for even one day. When the Lord led him to fast, it was by His might, one day at a time.

In the two years that I had been a Christian, I had heard about fasting. In my ignorance, I thought of it as nothing more than a work that people did to make themselves feel holier. However, an elder in my church, along with many others, began to enlighten me to fasting as a biblical principle of seeking God's face. He shared that in doing so, God's Spirit has been seen to move dramatically among His people. He challenged the church to fast and pray one Monday out of each month for revival in our lives and in our church.

In the past, I attempted to fast by my own strength. Upon self-examination, I found my underlying motive to be a selfish desire to lose weight. I always failed by dinner time. However, on February 25, 1996, God used a church elder to inspire me to pray about fasting for spiritual healing in our church and in my life. I prayed much of the next day as I fasted. I spoke with God, knowing I could do nothing without Him, that I desired to do His will and see Him glorified in my church, in my home, and in my life.

I felt so close to the Lord and so strong. Every day I would get up and ask if He wanted me to continue fasting. It just led to forty days. Every day I would pray about the church, the leadership, my family, and myself. I didn't feel weak in any way. I felt so spiritually revived. I was in the Word constantly and praying many times a day. Everything in my family and my life felt so connected. I was seeing changes in the church. The negative attitudes seemed to be replaced with an attitude of "what can we do?"

As a Christian, I knew I had a personal relationship with my Lord and Savior Jesus Christ. However, I found the joy of truly experiencing this relationship was in direct proportion to how much I took my eyes off myself and my surroundings and set them on the Lord Jesus and the needs of others. Time and time again, the Lord would direct me to Matthew 14:22–33 and the words Jesus said to Peter, "You of little faith, why did you doubt?" (v. 31). I realized how we must truly live by faith, and not by sight. My lapses of faith brought struggles with hunger in my fast, but when I put my complete trust in the Lord and His will, it was smooth sailing.

I had trouble at the very end because I took my eyes off the Lord, and focused more on achieving forty days. I likened it to Peter when he walked on the water. As soon as I put my eyes back on the Lord and asked Him to help me, when I focused on others with intercessory prayer, I saw things happening in answer to those prayers. I was amazed at what God was doing.

Since then I have to admit that, spiritually, it has been a decline. Gradually, but surely, I've gotten away from what I was doing during the fast—spending time with the Lord and praying. I didn't even realize that I had stopped reading and praying as often.

I tried to fast a few times after that and couldn't do it. That's why I know the forty-day fast was just something that God did in my life. It wasn't something I planned. He had planned it for me.

ॐ

You, too, will be blessed when God does a special, God-sized work through you. You will come to know Him in a way that will bring rejoicing to your life. When other people see you experiencing God that way, they are going to want to know how they, too, can experience God that way. Be prepared to point them to God...Pride may cause you to want to tell your experience because it makes you feel special. That will be a continuing tension. You will want to declare the wonderful deeds of the Lord, but you must avoid any sense of pride. Therefore: "He who glories, let him glory in the Lord" (1 Corinthians 1:31).

—Henry T. Blackaby and Claude V. King
Experiencing God

Evangelical Free Church

Louis G. Diaz is senior pastor of Evangelical Free Church of Wheaton, Illinois. His experiences show how fasting can help church leaders have a greater impact on individuals in their congregation.

Fasting has given me a greater awareness, an alert mind, keen senses, and a spiritual receptivity to what God is doing in my life and to see people as divine appointments. I've also experienced spiritual power in prayer—specific prayers for the healing of marriages and families. This heightened spiritual awareness has changed the way I deal with situations. For instance, one family was on the verge of breaking up. The wife and husband are solid Christians and, along with their children, are very involved in the church. They had been arguing, and she called me for emergency counseling. Previously, I would have scheduled counseling sessions for them, but I had a deeper understanding at that time. I suggested that we apply James 5:14 and the following verses to the marriage: "If anyone is sick, let him call for the elders."

The next day, the unheard-of happened. The wife, husband, and children were in my office. The elders gathered around the entire family. We told them we wanted to take a stand against the devil and the spiritual realm because we cared about them as a family. We anointed them with oil and prayed for the healing of the marriage. We told them that we wanted to lovingly hold them accountable, to make a difference in their marriage. I believe that the fast made me conscious of bringing God more into ministry than ever before. We followed that up with counseling and accountability sessions, and continue to seek to uplift them. This family now knows that you can turn to Jesus and to the spiritual leaders of the church.

The spiritual leaders are now going to get into homes and make a difference with families, not just have prayer meetings and share prayer requests but not get involved. I see that as a major difference. Prayer with personal involvement is more the direction we need to go.

I've also experienced power in preaching. One Sunday at the end of the message, I encouraged the congregation to take a stand right then that the standard of salvation is the holy character of God. Our church never asks people to stand or come forward, so this was very unusual. A huge number of people stood; many were weeping.

One Christian man had come that morning with his atheistic father-in-law who was visiting. He later told me that he didn't stand because he didn't want his father-in-law to feel uncomfortable. This young man felt convicted that he had denied Christ, just as Peter had denied Him. He told me, "I turned to my father-in-law who does not believe in God, and said to him, 'Dad, I should have stood. I just didn't want you to feel uncomfortable.'"

His father-in-law looked him straight in the eye and said, "When I heard the pastor's invitation to stand if you want to live a holy life for a holy God, I thought for sure you'd be the first one to stand."

This young man told me, "You keep calling us to holy living and standing for Jesus, because I will stand for Jesus no matter who is sitting around me. No matter what!"

God is calling me to activism for His kingdom by faith; to turn away from apathy; to stop being passive, tolerant, indifferent. It's a call to be *pro-active* for the kingdom by faith, and not *reactive*. I want to call God's people to influence the world.

We have heard that the witches and warlocks are fasting and praying for the demise of Christian leaders' homes. For a change, we are calling God's people to use this means of spiritual power for the kingdom and for fulfillment of the Great Commission.

❧

As long as you are proud you cannot know God...He
wants you to know Him: wants to give you Himself. And
He and you are two things of such a kind that if you really get into any kind of touch with Him you will, in fact, be
humble—delightedly humble, feeling the infinite relief of
having for once got rid of all the silly nonsense about
your own dignity which has made you restless and
unhappy all your life. He is trying to make you
humble in order to make this moment possible.

—C. S. Lewis
Mere Christianity

Citywide
Fasting and Prayer

What might happen if most of the churches in one area united to fast and pray for their city? This is the exciting adventure that many churches are discovering. As you will read in this section, the results are as varied as the areas in which the fasts occurred, but the stories are always miraculous.

Prayer for our communities is biblical. Moses (Exodus 32:31,32), Hezekiah (2 Kings 19:14–20), Daniel (Daniel 9:3–19), the king of Ninevah (Jonah 3:4–10), and many of the prophets prayed for their communities and nations and encouraged others to pray. Paul encourages us to pray against strongholds of spiritual wickedness (Ephesians 6:10–13) and to pray for the evangelization of those who need Jesus (Ephesians 6:18–20). He also exhorted believers to pray for all those in authority (1 Timothy 2:1,2). Our prayers will support and strengthen our pastor and church leaders.

I pray that these testimonies will encourage you to begin seeking God's face for your city or town. God can and will do a miraculous work in your area as you personally fast and pray, then unite with other Christians who have a similar burden to bring your churches and city before Him in intercessory prayer. As you do, God will begin moving in a new and wonderful way and will enable you to be channels of revival for your city.

Norfolk, Nebraska

Several citizens of Norfolk, Nebraska, saw God working through their prayer and fasting in extraordinary ways. Shelley Davy sent us her testimony and an article entitled, "40-Day Fasts Weakens Bodies, Strengthens Faith," from the Norfolk Daily News, *which reported on their experiences.*

It has been almost a year since the beginning of my forty-day fast. Since then, my husband and I have consistently set aside one day a week for fasting and prayer.

I am sending you a newspaper clipping about four more believers who were called to a forty-day fast. All completed it victoriously: Pastor Ron Gunsolley; Police Chief Bill Mizner and his wife, Kathy; and school board member Julee Pfeil:

> For five Norfolkans, this isn't a crazy story. It's reality. They all have completed a forty-day fast and they say their motivation was simple: a calling from God...
>
> But this was no planned thing. Although all four had visited with Mrs. Davy about her fast and the book she had read [*The Coming Revival*], they did not tell each other they planned to fast. It wasn't until each of them had started that they learned they were all fasting at the same time...
>
> "You may call it coincidental," Gunsolley said. "I would say we kind of think of it as providential that we were doing it at the same time. As we were discovering that we were doing it at the same time, it was a real good encouragement to share with each other what was going on and what was meaningful to each of us..."
>
> All five participants said the fast gave them humility and made them recognize their own human selfishness. Through the fast, they said, they learned to recognize how driven today's society is on consumption...
>
> Although such a fast involves a tremendous amount of sacrifice, the group said afterward they each felt an

enhanced spiritual life and deeper appreciation for life.

I sense God calling us to do a series of interviews on Christian radio explaining our reason for fasting.

∽

The experience of God's presence in those services was so real that at any moment I fully expected to hear the rustle of angels' wings. We saw amazing answers to prayer... All of the people who were prayed for in those services had been prayed for before, but when the family of God prayed together, there was an amazing and wonderful visitation of God. God was teaching us something important. He was teaching us to pray together; He was teaching us that He bends down low and listens to the sound of His people praying together.

—Steve Brown
Approaching God

Houston, Texas

It is thrilling to read how Christians in the Houston area took the initiative to bring together many believers to pray for revival. Not only did their efforts affect their city, but their ideas spread to other cities as well. This testimony comes from newsletter accounts of their fasting and prayer assemblies.

In January, Houston-area Christians completed forty days of fasting and prayer for revival. More than 10,000 people joined together from November 22, 1996, to January 1, 1997, every day and evening for intercession, evangelistic messages, corporate repentance, racial reconciliation, and praise and worship at "Prayer Mountain."

Earlier in 1996, Doug Stringer, founder of Turning Point Ministries, International, organized nearly two hundred churches of various denominations and ethnicity to reach Houston's poor, the gangs, the homeless, and the unsaved with an outreach called "Somebody Cares, Houston." As an outgrowth of their networking and cohesive efforts, they were prepared by the Holy Spirit for renewal. Stringer felt led of the Lord to present the idea of a forty-day citywide prayer effort to the pastors and leaders. Each one confirmed the direction from the Lord.

Stringer wrote to the Houston Christians:

> The Lord is drawing His Body together. This is the time; this is the hour to prepare for a move of God throughout our land…I believe the outpouring is due in part to the character of each of the men of God involved. These are men of character who have stood and wept between the porch and the altar for souls. God can entrust an outpouring to hearts prepared for such a visitation…A genuine passion for God allows no room for mediocrity. Any leaven in our hearts and lives must be purged so that we are totally consumed with a love for God and His truth. It is what we do behind closed doors where no one else can see us that determines the power of God or lack of it in public.[3]

While Houston's flat terrain doesn't offer much in the way of mountains, the Lord provided one. Doug Stringer met with the owner of a large outdoor amphitheater that is built at a high point overlooking the city. The owner agreed to rent the facility for forty days at a discounted rate. From late November to January 1, the facility was lovingly renamed "Prayer Mountain." Testimonies of how God provided every need—from the city waiving permit fees, to locating shuttle buses, to receiving funds from around the world to meet the costs—added to the confirmation that indeed this was His movement. More than three hundred pastors and ministry leaders met on Prayer Mountain on November 21 to unite in prayer and worship prior to the public meetings. A banner with the letters "P.U.S.H." was hung in front of the platform.

Doug Stringer writes:

> P.U.S.H.—Pray Until Something Happens—reminds us of a woman in labor. She is instructed to push. Push until something happens; pray until something happens. We believe that we are in the stage just before the birthing of a great move of God—an awakening that will impact not only Houston, but other parts of the world.[4]

Many expressed their deep appreciation at seeing the denominational and racial barriers falling down. Throughout the forty days, worship was led in Spanish, Korean, Chinese, Japanese, Indonesian, and many other languages. Messianic Jewish pastors publicly embraced Arab ministers; Chinese and Japanese leaders prayed for one another; walls between people fell as they worshipped the Lord in unity.

Lives were changed in miraculous ways as well. "I was involved in gangs," a 19-year-old man explained, "and two months ago was released from prison. A friend of mine invited me to come to Prayer Mountain tonight. Jesus saved me." This man now wants to train for ministry. Numerous stories of healings even of cancer and blindness, deliverance from addictions including crack cocaine, renewed marriages, and family healing were reported. Many expressed a renewed and deepened love for the Lord.

Each day at six in the morning, at noon, and at least three hours each evening, corporate prayer and evangelism services were held at the amphitheater. In addition, on December 7 a benevolence ministry reaching out to those in need distributed enough groceries for 5,000 needy families through Operation Blessing; clothes, blankets, food, and toys were given to 600 children for Christmas. GOAD International also provided 40,000 pounds of food and 1,000 blankets for distribution.

Turning Point Ministries, International collected prayer requests that were read during the services, enabling God to melt cold hearts.

"I want us to feel the pain, the hurt, the desperation," Stringer said, "of parents, children, husbands, wives, the lonely, the sick who need healing, so it's no longer just sympathy, but true empathy—identifying." Stringer also spoke of what it means to humble ourselves before the Lord. "Old wineskins are going to have to go. God is saying 'new wineskins' for what He wants to do, but let God do it His way and not ours. We have to be led of the Spirit, and sometimes that means a lot of death in our own ideas and our own ways of doing things. One of our statements at Turning Point Ministries, International, is: 'While men reach for thrones to build their own kingdoms, Jesus reached for a towel to wash men's feet.' We must maintain a posture of humility and servanthood if we are to see a genuine move of God."

> *We must maintain a posture of humility and servanthood if we are to see a genuine move of God.*

Claire Greiner, youth pastor at Houston's Glorious Way Church, writes, "People streamed to the altar every night, eager to get into a right relationship with God. Those who had before tried to pick specks out of the eyes of others were challenged to pull the planks out of their own... God's searchlight shone on hearts, and in His light, people caught glimpses of the holy nature of God Himself."[5]

Deborah DeGar, founder of International Prayer Fellowship School of Prayer, explained the importance of Houston's renewal. "God dealt with the fact that we have an exterior that says we're Christians, but in our actions nobody can tell the difference between us and the world in our workplaces and the various places that we go. God is pulling off the mask." DeGar believes God is preparing

Houston for His work. "We couldn't move into it until He worked with our hearts to break them, to circumcise them, to bring us to a place of repentance, so that the purity of the revival can come forth. Every night was a different purging."[6]

On January 1, Houston symbolically passed the baton to Dallas. On January 3, Dallas Christians began forty days of fasting and prayer for their city. In February, believers in both Kansas City and Pasadena, California, started their forty-day, citywide fasting and prayer. At this writing, nine cities have agreed to participate in consecutive forty-day periods of fasting and prayer around the country, and many more are considering joining as well!

⤳

If the sinless Christ, who is literally God in human flesh and Lord of all, would so humble Himself for us, we dare not denigrate humility or aspire to self-esteem instead of lowliness...Do you want to be blessed? Develop a servant's heart. If Jesus can step down from His glorious equality with God to become a man, and then further humble Himself to be a servant and wash the feet of twelve undeserving sinners—then humble Himself to die so horribly on our behalf, surely we ought to be willing to suffer any indignity to serve Him.

John MacArthur
"Humility," *Moody Magazine*

Dallas/Ft. Worth, Texas

At our last inquiry, nearly 2,500 people had registered to complete a forty-day fast. Others had agreed to participate in a partial or part-time fast, as well. More than 120 pastors and their churches are involved in this citywide fast. Pastor Byron Mote of Eaglemount Family Church has taken on the responsibility of orchestrating this effort. My staff and I look forward to hearing about the great things God is doing in Texas.

Pastor Mote was impressed with the Houston fast and felt led of the Lord to take it to the Dallas area immediately. Their fast began on January 3. A group of twenty pastors who met weekly agreed with his vision. They, in turn, called pastors citywide to join them.

Hundreds of copies of *The Coming Revival* were distributed throughout the area to guide people on the vision and the process of a juice fast. The Lord has given these pastors a vision of thousands of young people being saved and businesses so consumed with revival that regular work would need to be suspended for a time.

Midway through the fast, Pastor Mote commented on the citywide fast. "The main result is in the area of holiness. God is severely dealing with all of us about the little foxes in our lives."

A fax and E-mail system was established to "receive any dreams, visions, or prophetic words that God may reveal to people during their forty days of prayer and fasting. These will be judged scripturally as best we can and the major ones submitted to…Bill Bright's office."

⌇⌇

The general statement, "The effectual, fervent prayer of a righteous man availeth much," is a statement of prayer as an energetic force. Two words are used. One signifies power in exercise, operative power, while the other is power as an endowment. Prayer is power and strength, a power and strength which influences God, and is most salutary, widespread, and marvelous in its gracious benefits to man.

—E. M. Bounds
The Possibilities of Prayer

Colorado Springs, Colorado

Forty-three Colorado Springs pastors, leaders, and spouses participated in a forty-day fast in the fall of 1996. While not a "city-

wide" fast in that it was not open to everyone, it still encompassed a vast number of churches and parachurch organizations. It crossed denominational and ethnic lines and brought together some of the most influential minds in the evangelical world. Mr. Jaan Heinmets, Campus Crusade for Christ staff member in Colorado Springs, gave details of the group fast.

More than sixty churches were involved in the fast, most for the entire forty days. It impacted our city with a spirit of unity that is much stronger than before. We sought to utilize our differences for the Body of Christ, rather than diminish or work around them. Perhaps for the first time, lay people now hear their pastor praying for the pastor of another church in this city. This has inspired a greater spirit of unity, not competition.

Our fast, begun in October, was planned to end on the last day of the Fasting & Prayer '96 gathering in St. Louis. More than one hundred people from Colorado Springs attended the St. Louis conference. We sensed that God was going to do something mighty in our city, and it would spread from the leadership down.

One of the efforts that grew out of our fasting together was the launch of a twenty-four-hour prayer vigil called "Love Colorado Springs." Beginning on Valentine's Day, February 14, 1997, churches and parachurch organizations will take one day a month to pray for the city.

We are seeking to love our city and see God's blessings poured out on Colorado Springs. In this way, we will show each other, as well as the city, our unity and love.

⁓

Devote yourselves to prayer, being watchful and thankful. And pray for us, too, that God may open a door for our message, so that we may proclaim the mystery of Christ, for which I am in chains. Pray that I may proclaim it clearly, as I should. Be wise in the way you act toward outsiders;

> make the most of every opportunity. Let your conversation
> be always full of grace, seasoned with salt, so that
> you may know how to answer everyone.
>
> —Colossians 4:2–6

Pueblo, Colorado

Dr. Curt Dodd is pastor of the Fellowship of the Rockies church in Pueblo. His stirring testimony tells of the battles Christians face in this city.

As you know, there are many Christian organizations that have made Colorado Springs their headquarters. There are probably more Christians per capita there than anywhere in the United States. However, just thirty-eight miles south, Pueblo lies in spiritual darkness as less than five percent of its population attends church.

As an example of what we face in Pueblo, a young lady came to our town to start the universal church of Wicca (witches) saying that her spiritual advisors had led her to pick Pueblo as the most ripe place to begin a work. In fact, one of the people won to Christ through our church came out of the occult. He told me that people come from all over to receive "special energy" radiated in Pueblo.

In December 1995, God impressed us to begin the new year with an extended time of prayer and fasting for the breaking of the darkness over Pueblo. I called the president of Pueblo's association of evangelical Christian leaders and inquired if any plans had been made concerning such a call. He told me that through the efforts of a church layman, the city council had just passed a proclamation calling for January 2 through February 10, 1996, to be set aside as forty days of prayer and fasting to break the darkness over this town.

If you only knew what a miracle that is in itself! The next day one of our pastors was talking to a lady from a Lutheran church who had just come back from a retreat. Her testimony was, "God has impressed on us that we are to begin praying and fasting to break the darkness in this place." Like us, she and her church did not know of the city council's decision, nor of the quiet harmony that God was orchestrating.

I have studied spiritual awakenings for years, and since my seminary days have prayed that I could be part of such a movement of God. Great awakenings are not the result of great organization or even great preaching, but simple, fervent fasting and prayer on the part of God's people.

※

> If we obey God, it is going to cost other people more than it costs us, and that is where the sting comes in. If we are in love with our Lord, obedience does not cost us anything, it is a delight, but it costs those who do not love Him a good deal. If we obey God, it will mean that other people's plans are upset, and they will gibe [ridicule] us with it— "You call this Christianity?" We can prevent the suffering; but if we are going to obey God, we must not prevent it, we must let the cost be paid.
>
> —Oswald Chambers
> *My Utmost for His Highest*

Hacienda Heights, California

Frederic Chen is the senior pastor at United Christian Church in Hacienda Heights, California. After reading The Coming Revival, *he and his wife were prompted to fast and pray for forty days. Their commitment inspired them to encourage others to join them in fasting.*

Through our fasting and prayer, we learned so much from our Lord. We have received many spiritual and physical blessings.

We wanted to share our blessings, so we encouraged the people in our church concerning fasting and praying. On September 1, 1995, we began a 100 Days of Fasting and Prayer relay within our own congregation. Hundreds in our congregation are fasting and praying for various amounts of time in the next one hundred days. We praise God for this encouragement and confirmation of His work.

I am part of the Holy Spirit Renewal Fellowship. This is a group of Chinese pastors and their wives in East Los Angeles County who meet monthly. The Spirit has also moved among them. Now many of them have begun their forty days of fasting and prayer as well.

We distributed more than three hundred copies of *The Coming Revival* in this area. I am trusting in the Lord that He is doing a mighty work in the Chinese churches. I know that there will be many Chinese Christians who will be among the two million that you are praying for who will pray and fast for the revival of the country and for the world.

⤳

The important thing for us as Christians is not what we eat or drink but stirring up goodness and peace and joy from the Holy Spirit. If you let Christ be Lord in these affairs, God will be glad; and so will others. In this way aim for harmony in the church and try to build each other up.

—Romans 14:17–19 (TLB)

Enid, Oklahoma

Rob Cummins sent this letter about how he shared prayer videos with a local pastor, which helped spark a citywide fasting and prayer effort. Rob is enthused about the results.

I attended both Fasting and Prayer '95 and '96 and will continue to participate in every such gathering. In my twenty years as a Christian, these were the most important investments I have ever made in the kingdom. When I read *The Coming Revival,* I immediately sensed that this was God's heart. Since then I have been promoting prayer for revival in our community. I am not normally that outgoing, but I simply feel that I must share what God has placed on my heart.

Sharing my experience with a local pastor and showing him Concerts of Prayer's video *Get Ready for the Coming Revival* proved to be a catalyst to promote revival prayer among local leaders. A group of pastors and lay leaders now fast and pray together on Mondays. The mix in this group would suggest that the prayer movement in our city is crossing ethnic and denominational boundaries.

This weekly prayer time, in turn, has spilled over into a monthly gathering that is evolving into a mini Concert of Prayer. In this core group, there is an effort to organize a citywide Concert of Prayer that coincides with the National Day of Prayer. We are also planning to have a satellite link in Enid for Prayer and Fasting '97. I think it is fair to say that much of this prayer can be traced to Dr. Bright's book and to the Fasting & Prayer gatherings of '95 and '96.

> *Whereas I once thought the battlefield was "out there" among those who are rejecting Christ, I see things differently now... The front-line of the battle is in the hearts of God's people.*

Becoming more vocal about God's conditional plans for America and the idea that those plans hinge on an appropriate response of humility by God's people has definitely exposed me to a spiritual battle. Whereas I once thought the battlefield was primarily "out there" among those who are rejecting Christ, I see things differently now. I honestly feel the front-line of the battle is in the hearts of God's people.

It is very sobering to find how many people whom I would presume to be saved feel little or no urgency regarding their spiritual condition, the condition of the church, or that of our nation. The prevailing mood of many seems to be that things are not really so bad. I also encounter a sense of hopelessness and futility, which I think is born out of unbelief. I get easily discouraged when I encounter this, but I am persuaded that God is speaking to His Church that He is getting ready to do something the likes of which we have never seen, and that it is time to get ready.

~

It is my pleasure to tell you about the miraculous signs and wonders that the Most High God has performed for me. How great are his signs, how mighty his wonders! His kingdom is an eternal kingdom; his dominion endures from generation to generation.

—Daniel 4:2,3

Katy, Texas

Located just outside of Houston, the city of Katy also got involved in the fasting and prayer movement. The "domino effect" of one fast produced amazing results!

After reading *The Coming Revival,* Dr. Charles J. Wisdom, pastor of First Baptist Church, completed a fifteen-day fast. During his regularly scheduled meeting with several other pastors of the city, Dr. Wisdom spoke about making prayer and fasting a part of their church efforts. The pastors then decided to ask the mayor of Katy to declare a forty-day fast for the entire city.

In conjunction with the May 2 National Day of Prayer, the mayor, a committed Christian, and the city council agreed to declare Forty Days of Prayer and Fasting in Katy from May 2 to June 10. A formal proclamation appeared in the local newspaper inviting all citizens to participate.

(The proclamation and newspaper advertising are reprinted in Appendix E.)

They also listed suggested levels of participation which included a variety of prayer efforts, as well as fasting choices that ranged from one meal a day for forty days up to the full forty-day fast. People who could not fast from food were encouraged to fast from some other pleasure such as television.

The Pastor's Prayer Fellowship organized citywide, interdenominational prayer services during the declared forty-day fast. Throughout the city, coworkers, neighbors, students, and other associations organized their own prayer groups that met regularly during that period.

"We were asking God to visit our city," Dr. Wisdom explains. "We are very encouraged by what we have seen. An important seed was planted and has taken root. I believe a harvest of the cross has been demonstrated by our fasting and prayer. Our Pastor's Fellowship has already informed the mayor that we are building on this for another forty-day fast next May."

During the fast, many people met on Tuesdays at 5 a.m. and at noon on Wednesdays to pray for the city. Even after the fast, people continue to meet at those times for prayer. The momentum continues to build for a great work of God in Katy resulting from their citywide fast.

﹏

An interesting similarity exists between feeling the loss of a loved one who has died and the conviction of sin and repentance in the Bible. Both involve mourning. Brokenness is similar to both of these events. The death of a dream hurts. If you are like Uncle Remus singing "Zippidy Doo Da," you are not experiencing brokenness. Even as you become aware of what needs to happen in your life, relinquishing selfishness, submitting your goals,

or surrendering your rights, you still feel a sense of
loss in your life. A part of yourself is being put to
death, even a loathsome, fruitless part.

—Alan E. Nelson
Broken in the Right Place

Kent, Washington

Frank Zvonec and his wife are lay people with a teaching ministry called Morning Star Ministries. Frank describes how he shared his experiences of fasting and prayer with others.

In October 1993, the Lord instructed me to call groups of believers together to pray and fast for three days. Thus far, we have held four such gatherings here in the Northwest, and each one seems to get better. The Lord has provided large conference grounds for all these events at virtually no cost, and His glorious presence has transformed many lives. In March 1994, more than ninety people from forty-three churches came together for a water-only fast. This past March, seventy-eight of us broke the three-day fast with worship and the Lord's supper. It was a very precious moment that I'll never forget.

Can you envision what God might do if millions of Christians would shut off their televisions for forty days and cry out to Him?

God has shown me that He honors all types of prayer and fasting when done with pure motives and a repentant heart. I recently contacted several pastors and challenged them to fast from television for forty days and to ask their congregations to do the same. Can you envision what God might do if millions of Christians would shut off their televisions for forty days and cry out to Him?

I recently completed a forty-day "Daniel fast" in which I had only fruit, vegetables, and water. There was nothing spectacular in the first thirty days, but the results were very powerful. Like many men, I often struggled with impatience and a bad attitude while driving. The Lord has been dealing with me in this area for many years. On the thirty-fifth day of my fast, I confessed this sin (again) and forsook it. I had great confidence that God was pleased and would answer, and He did. I have experienced an incredible breakthrough in this area of my life.

۞

The Lord says he who formed me in the womb to be his servant to bring Jacob back to Him and gather Israel to himself, for I am honored in the eyes of the Lord and my God has been my strength—he says: "It is too small a thing for you to be my servant to restore the tribes of Jacob and bring back those of Israel I have kept. I will also make you a light for the Gentiles, that you may bring my salvation to the ends of the earth."

—Isaiah 49:5,6

Modesto, California

Many are calling the spiritual change in this area "the miracle in Modesto." Reverend Glenn Barteau, pastor of Calvary Temple Worship Center, and Reverend David Seifert, pastor of Big Valley Grace Community Church, describe some examples of a spiritual awakening in Modesto that has changed lives in the churches and in the community. Following a Christian drama, Heaven's Gates, Hell's Flames, *thousands of people responded to the gospel.*

Individuals, as well as entire families, have been changed tremendously. Thousands of children have received the Lord. More than ten thousand teenagers have given their lives to the Lord. Young people who were in gangs brought their "colors" and their "rags" and said, "I'm not going to be in a gang anymore."

The Lord was working in all spectrums of people—from both sides of the track, rich and poor, those who were doing well in their lives and those who weren't. It was an outpouring on every person in our area, and it was just an unbelievable move of God.

We're confident that this began in the throne room of God. Matthew Henry said that when God intends great mercy for His people, He calls them to prayer. It began a couple of years ago when our church leaders went on a four-day, no-agenda prayer summit. The goal was to seek God and say, "Lord, what do you want to do in us?" We're so used to doing our own programs and our own agenda that it was very difficult for us, but in the process God bound our hearts together and gave us a love for each other. We began to realize that God puts His blessing on people of unity. He does not bless just any kind of unity, but the kind that Jesus prayed in John 17:11, asking that all who believe in Him would be one.

From that summit and our convictions for unity, we began to pray together weekly in the business center of our town. For more than a year, over fifty pastors have gathered every Wednesday to pray and seek God's face.

God prepares a congregation by preparing the pastor and the leadership. We prepared by having a forty-day fast. We had hundreds of people fasting every day for forty days. Then, the week before the drama came to the church, we had a three-day fast. Every member of the church was asked to write the names of unsaved people and lay those names on the altar in our sanctuary. At noon for three days, we'd go to the altar and hold those names as we prayed for each person. We entered into intense spiritual warfare in prayer.

Of course, it took a lot of work in all areas, a lot of organization. Even so, the blessings of God were far beyond what we could ever have imagined. God visited our city! When God moves, people take on a whole new nature—God's nature. We were saying, "God, as You're pulling us, we're just trying to hang on. Our feet are barely touching the ground. We just want to keep up with You."

To see thousands come to God, to see the church altars filled every night—often with unchurched people—was phenomenal!

This drama, *Heaven's Gates and Hell's Flames*, speaks to people about hope. America has a whole generation that lacks hope. They're futureless, they're directionless, they're trying to survive day by day. Everybody's trying to find something that they can hold on to. This play dealt with the separation from loved ones that so many people experience today.

> *Matthew Henry said that when God intends great mercy for His people, He calls them to prayer.*

A young boy who was a gang member in Stockton came to the altar, and he had on his hat, his gang gear. His mom was standing with him. The pastor at the front asked him, "Son, why did you come forward? Why do you want to get saved?" He said, "My grandmother died about two weeks ago, and she was a Christian. Well, I want to see her again, and I realize if I don't get saved, I won't ever see my grandmother again." So, the aspect of separation speaks to many people.

Four generations of one family came forward and received Christ—a little girl six years old, her mother, grandmother, and great-grandmother.

Thirty-three thousand people signed commitment cards indicating that they have received Christ. We did not know how we could follow up on that kind of a harvest. It becomes overwhelming. Yet throughout this year, thousands of them have been baptized and have become a part of our fellowship.

All the churches in the area banded together in this effort. They received cards on individuals to call them and try to network with their family members. This spiritual harvest also affected the workplace in Modesto. We have prayed that Christian men and women would begin to openly share their faith and truly love and pray for unbelievers around them. We have heard many stories of how God has answered our prayers.

The special emphasis on fasting and prayer, along with continued prayer on a regular basis by the pastors of this community, have changed Modesto. God has met us here in a gracious and abundant way.

ᔰ

> The great work of intercession is needed for this returning to the Lord. It is here that the coming revival must find its strength...Let there be, with every minister and worker, "great searchings of heart" (Judges 5:16), as to whether they are ready to give as much time and strength to prayer as God desires. Let them, even as they are, in public, leaders of their larger or smaller circles, give themselves, in secret, to take their places in the front rank of the great intercession host.
>
> —Andrew Murray
> *The Ministry of Intercession*

Reno, Nevada

Reno, Nevada, is known around the world as "Sin City." Only five percent of the population attends church on Sunday. Yet the vision of one pastor for revival, a new unity among the churches, and ministry direction has now gripped the city. Pastor Jim Wallace, who serves at Northgate Community Church in the neighboring community of Sparks, participated in a united effort by area churches to fast and pray for Reno. He believes it was no coincidence that the revival followed on the heels of the first Fasting & Prayer gathering in Orlando.

"In late August and early September 1995," Pastor Wallace explained, "God began to speak to me about prayer and revival. I immediately wrote a letter to the other pastors in the area encouraging them to begin joining together to pray seriously for revival.

"In May 1996, a friend, Pastor Jim Krupa, and I went on a seven-day fast. God answered our prayers for unity among churches in our area and for direction with regard to revival in a remarkable and supernatural way. We became convinced that we needed to put feet to our prayers and call God's people, the Church, to repentance in 1997. We became convinced that the glory cloud of His manifest presence would descend upon Reno if His people properly prepared themselves to receive it. The proper preparation? Prayer, fasting, repentance."

Pastors Wallace and Krupa met with sixty pastors—across denominational lines—at a Strategy Summit to reach Reno for Christ by the year 2000. Several pastors began to meet weekly for prayer and renewal within the Body of Christ. They knew of the examples of Moses and John the Baptist calling the people to repentance before God came to them. The churches of Reno would also need to prepare themselves if they wanted God to change their city

They designated a citywide forty-day fast from January 13 to February 21, 1997. The fast could be from food (a juice fast) or from other things. Even children agreed to fast from television, candy, or rock music. Twenty-two churches committed to the fast. The churches agreed to hold a special time of prayer each Sunday afternoon for all participants to meet together. The location was rotated among the participating churches.

The day after the fast ended (Saturday, February 22), everyone met for a half-day at their own churches. In the evening, a joint celebration of prayer and praise was held.

The weekly prayer sessions between pastors continue, along with a special emphasis in the churches to pray for the city. A November 8 Sacred Assembly is being planned. This is based on the passage in Joel 1 where God calls for a public fast. That will be a day of seeking God's face in fasting and prayer. Government and public officials will be invited to attend as well.

Pastor Wallace asks, "Please be praying that the united Christians of Reno will come together in prevailing prayer and that we will recognize the woe due to our city because of the greatness of our sin. And pray that there will truly be a repentance among God's people that will result in a great awakening in this place which so desperately needs God's grace!"

∽

"Your attitude toward me has been proud and arrogant," says the Lord. "But you say, 'What do you mean? What have we said that we shouldn't?' "Listen; you have said, 'It is foolish to worship God and obey him. What good does it do to obey his laws, and to sorrow and mourn for our sins? From now on, as far as we're concerned, "Blessed are the arrogant." For those who do evil shall prosper, and those who dare God to punish them shall get off scot-free.'" Then those who feared and loved the Lord spoke often of him to each other. And he had a Book of Remembrance drawn up in which he recorded the names of those who feared him and loved to think about Him. "They shall be mine," says the Lord Almighty, "in that day when I make up my jewels. And I will spare them as a man spares an obedient and dutiful son. Then you will see the difference between God's treatment of good men and bad, between those who serve him and those who don't."

—Malachi 3:13–18 (TLB)

Bakersfield, California

Dr. David Goh of Bakersfield Community Church, located two hours north of Los Angeles, has joined with six other church lead-

ers to call this community to fast, pray, and seek God's face for the
forty days prior to Palm Sunday, 1997. The churches represent
African-American, Asian, Hispanic, and Anglo races, and six
different denominations.

The pastors sent a "Call to Prayer" invitation throughout the city. This brochure explains that this fast is for "*renewal* for every congregation in our city (in whatever manner appropriate for their tradition and expression) and *unity* for us as the one Body of Christ; *justice and provision* for the economically, socially, and educationally deprived; *reconciliation and freedom* from the strongholds of evil that manifest themselves through drug and alcohol abuse, gang and domestic violence, poverty, pornography, family disintegration, child abuse, and abortion; and *citywide revival,* which will result in thousands accepting Christ *in* our city and many people sent *from* our city to fulfill the Great Commission throughout the world."

The mayor of the city is releasing a call to repentance to begin the Lenten season with special activities planned for the community. Fifty-seven churches are enlisted to participate in some way during the fast.

Leslie Barnes sent us a report on the Bakersfield fast, in which she says:

> Several of my churchmates and my pastor have been greatly stimulated and encouraged through reading your book on *The Coming Revival.*
>
> You may already know that a multi-racial, multi-denominational group of pastors and Christian laymen have taken to heart your call to fast and pray and have called for a forty-day fast and prayer time for the Christians of Bakersfield. Around 80–100 churches are participating in this in one form or another. The mayor made a proclamation, and TV spots on 2 Chronicles 7:14 have aired. We are encouraged at what God is doing and at seeing this many churches working and uniting in prayer together.

ॐ

The very thing that the church professes to have,
namely love and acceptance, is often the thing that
is flagrantly lacking among its own members.

—Luci Swindoll
The Alchemy of the Heart

Spokane, Washington

This testimony shows how God is moving among churches in one area. The leadership in the Spokane area took the initiative in promoting fasting and prayer with great success. I am sure that God will bless their efforts.

A call went out to 722 churches in the Inland Northwest inviting them to participate in a fast from February 17 to March 28, 1997. The leadership plans to show videos of the satellite program of the Fasting & Prayer '96 gathering in St. Louis. The fast will include prayer vigils from Friday night through Saturday morning and will conclude with a solemn assembly on Good Friday. In addition, morning prayer meetings will be held at different sites throughout the area.

Forty Spokane pastors have been meeting for prayer, and much reconciliation has already occurred across the city. A one-day seminar was held to help people understand fasting and prayer and revival, followed by an evening of worship and renewal.

At this time, more than sixty churches have agreed to participate in the forty-day fast.

ॐ

Fasting produces spiritual introspection, spiritual
examination, spiritual confession, and spiritual intercession.

—Elmer L. Towns
Fasting for Spiritual Breakthrough

Nationwide Fasting and Prayer

In talking with many prominent Christian leaders across our land, I have witnessed a growing concern for the tragic condition of America. It is obvious that the Holy Spirit has been at work among those who will listen to His voice, and that He is creating this concern in the minds and hearts of His people. This is demonstrated by the testimonies in this section. You will read of the creative ways Christians are spreading information about fasting and prayer and the results of their national efforts.

Also included is a story about how God is working on the college campus. All over this country in Christian colleges and secular universities, repentance, confession, and renewal have been flourishing since 1995. Starting with the Brownwood, Texas, church and nearby Payne University, the fire spread to Illinois, Massachusetts, Kentucky, Florida, and on and on. Churches near many of these colleges broke out in repentance and a new experience of the Holy Spirit. To me, it appears more than happenstance that God would begin to answer the prayers of His children so shortly after the Orlando Fasting & Prayer gathering on December 4–6, 1994.

I encourage you to read further about this incredible work of God in *Revival!* by John Avant, Malcolm McDow, and Alvin Reid, and in *Accounts of a Campus Revival: Wheaton College*, edited by Timothy Beougher and Lyle Dorsett.

Perhaps you know of or are involved in a fasting and prayer effort that has national coverage. I would love to hear about your experiences. I also encourage you to search for nationwide fasting and prayer efforts in your area.

National fasting and prayer gatherings are co-sponsored annually by Campus Crusade for Christ and Mission America. Key Christian leaders and thousands of laypersons convene for the conference and millions more participate via satellite. For more information, call (888) 327-8464.

Dr. Ronnie Floyd

Dr. Ronnie Floyd, a well-known speaker, is chairman of the executive committee of the Southern Baptist Convention and author of several books, including The Meaning of a Man: Discovering Your Destiny as a Spiritual Champion. *He also is pastor of First Baptist Church in Springdale, Arkansas. He gave the opening call to worship at the St. Louis Fasting & Prayer '96 gathering (his address is reprinted in Appendix B). His testimony is an inspiring example of how God is moving among people all over our nation.*

Early one morning in March 1995, the Lord spoke to me through His Word, calling me to a forty-day period of fasting and prayer for the purpose of seeing revival in America, in my church, and in my life. Even though I have practiced fasting for years, this was an unusual call of God. As I struggled to obey, I determined that it was the will of God. The next Sunday, someone laid on my desk a copy of Dr. Bright's book *The Coming Revival.* What God had done through him was unknown to me, but served as a confirmation that God was up to something. His book became the practical advice to me concerning a prolonged fast.

After forty days of being with God that radically transformed my life and ministry, the Lord gave me the freedom to share my journey with my 9,000-member church. As a result, God came on that Sunday morning. On June 4, 1995, I saw the greatest movement of God that I had ever seen up to that point in my life. Our morning worship service lasted two-and-a-half hours and was filled with the holiness of God and deep spiritual brokenness. Seventy percent of the crowd returned on Sunday evening, and our worship service lasted for more than four hours. I saw weeping, wailing, repentance, restoration of relationships, open confession of sin, and healing of all kinds. God came. Since that day, our church has never been the same.

Out of this forty-day fast, God called me to travel across the country with a worship team and band, holding "Awaken America Rallies." These one-night rallies are calling the people of God to repentance and to revival principles like prayer and fasting. In the first year, we have been in almost twenty cities across the land.

In addition, the Lord led me to write the book *The Meaning of a Man*. The book gives testimony about this fast, but has a passion to call men to revival by becoming what they need to become. Released in April 1996, the book is already in its fourth printing.

At the 1995 Pastors' Conference of the Southern Baptist Convention, I gave testimony through my preaching about this forty-day fast. God has used it to make the entire denomination aware of this ministry—which we all need to be a part of as Christians. Many have responded by getting with God for forty days. In my own church, at least twenty laypersons have successfully completed a forty-day period of fasting and prayer.

In February 1996, the Lord began to call me to another forty-day fast, and I submitted to His leadership in March. Revival was again the passion that God put on my heart.

The Lord led me to share this journey with my church. Once again, the Holy Spirit poured out great blessings as our worship service on Sunday morning lasted almost three hours. An unbelievable mighty move of God took place.

On June 10, 1996, I preached to the Pastors' Conference of the Southern Baptist Convention on "God's Gateway to Supernatural Power." This message was a call to humble ourselves before God through prayer and fasting. It was the first time that I know of that anyone addressed the group solely on this subject. Thousands heard the message and are responding in fasting and prayer.

On June 12, I preached the keynote convention sermon. I challenged the audience about spiritual leadership, calling them to prayer, fasting, and repentance, as well as sharing with them about the revival of the Holy Spirit that will be sent before the coming of Jesus. I concluded the message by doing something that no one had ever done in this setting: I felt God was leading me to challenge us as pastors of the entire Southern Baptist Convention of 40,000 churches and 16 million members to do the following:

> On October 27, 1996, in the morning church service, preach on the subject of fasting, calling our people to observe October 30 as a day of humiliation, prayer, and fasting. In the evening service lead our churches in a solemn assembly, a time when we cry out to God over our sins and the sins of our nation, begging for the mercy of God to come upon us. On October 30 observe a day of fasting, prayer, and humiliation, for the purpose of seeing revival personally, in our churches, in our denomination, and in America. On November 3 preach in the morning and evening services on the subject of spiritual revival, calling the people to it, regardless of the cost.

At the conclusion of the message, thousands of people responded. The Spirit fell. It was an unbelievable experience for each of us. So many had prayed for this for years.

I had the privilege of sharing about this emphasis on the "700 Club" television program with Pat Robertson in July, to 10,000 people at Jerry Falwell's Super Conference, and on James Dobson's "Focus on the Family" radio broadcast. Hopefully, this emphasis will transcend denominational lines. God is moving; He is up to something.

We are currently having a prayer revival in our church. Several of our lay people have undergone a forty-day fast. I have a group of men who cover me with prayer and fasting every day of every week. There's not one day that our church is not in prayer and fasting. They call themselves "The Pastor's Mighty Men," and it's one of the greatest gifts I've ever been given.

Prayer and fasting has revolutionized my life and ministry. God has given me a life message that is being shared around the world. All of this has happened as a result of obedience to God in my life: Obedience to prayer and fasting, then obedience to do what He has called me to do in it. Praise His holy name.

✌

If we embrace a self-absorbed hedonism of relaxation and happy feelings, while dodging tough tasks, unpopular stances and exhausting relationships—we fall short of the biblical God-centeredness and the cross-bearing life to which Jesus calls us, and advertise to the world nothing better than our own decadence.

—J. I. Packer
Hot Tub Religion

Max Lucado

My dear friend Max Lucado presented a challenge to Christians to fast and pray for the forty days prior to the 1996 presidential election, calling it "Forty Days of Faith." Over 40,000 people responded to the call! Max is pastor of Oak Hills Church of Christ in San Antonio, Texas, and is an author and radio speaker.

The purpose of the challenge of "Forty Days of Faith," Rev. Lucado writes, was to "pray for God to have His way with America—not an effort to promote a candidate, party, or opinion. We were simply asking God to shine His face on America."

Prayer partners were asked to make a commitment to pray daily following a specific prayer guide, and to fast one time for a period of their own choosing during the forty days from September 27 to November 5, 1996.

"Forty Days of Faith" was launched on the radio program *UpWords*. Originally, the goal was to reach 10,000 people to pray and fast. The overwhelming response of more than 40,000 was totally unexpected. "Prayer partners from coast to coast have begged God to have mercy upon this nation and guide us in our election," writes Lucado. "If my math is correct, then over a million prayers have been offered during these forty days! We can be confident that, because we prayed, the world is different today than it would have been had we not prayed.

"May God bring a holy shake-up. May He shake us loose from sins. Nineteenth-century preacher Charles Spurgeon prayed that God would give His church a season of 'glorious disorder'—not a disorder that means chaos, but a disorder that startles us into alertness, awakening us to the need for revival in our land. Prayer does not always lead to revival, but revival always follows prayer."

ॐ

Blessed is the man who endures temptation; for when he has been proved, he will receive the crown of life which the Lord has promised to those who love Him.

—James 1:12 (NKJ)

Laurie Killingsworth

Laurie is the national coordinator and speaker for Passionate Hearts, a retreat ministry for women to bring them into personal revival and intimacy with God. He clearly gave her the vision to begin this ministry in 1994, and the first retreat was held in 1995. She is so excited about how women are praying to receive

Christ, beginning to fast, and agreeing to pray in triplets. Laurie, who lives in Orlando, Florida, tells how fasting has made a difference in her life.

As I sit down to write the impact that prayer with fasting has had in my life and ministry over the past two years, I am at a loss to summarize it! How can I explain what it means to have intimacy with God and input from Him on a daily basis that I only experienced intermittently during my previous twenty-five years in ministry? How can I explain how the Spirit is as close as my breath? How can I explain His ways of giving a vision and then clarifying it over and over again? How can I explain a continual flow of answered prayer? All I can do is give a few broad strokes and highlights and pray that He will somehow use it in someone's life as a challenge to take Him at His word, obey Him by faith, and move forward step-by-step in obedience.

In the days that followed the December 1994 Orlando Fasting & Prayer gathering, God began to open a clear vision to me of launching a women's retreat ministry, *Passionate Hearts,* to call women in the churches to revival —to walk in power, purity, and prayer with fasting. Within two months, I'd spoken at two women's retreats. The response at both was the same and has continued in all subsequent retreats: an average of 26 percent receive Christ, 63 percent surrender to the Holy Spirit's control, 70 percent commit themselves to a weekly prayer triplet, and 45 percent commit to fasting with their prayer life!

It wasn't until April 3, 1996, however, that I felt a strong leading into a forty-day fast. The call was certain, and four days later, on Easter night, I began. (A day later, my dear husband, Tip, joined me for the duration!) That forty days was the best of all worlds and the worst of all worlds! It was *not* easy and the warfare was intense at times, but I believe the results will last not just for a lifetime, but for eternity.

The very clear theme that jumped out at me was that throughout Scripture, the number 40 is related to the principle that after discipline and suffering comes God's provision, promise, and completion.

On day forty of my fast, revival broke out during a *Passionate Hearts* retreat at a mainline denominational church in Ft. Lauderdale, Florida, after my first message on Friday evening called "Women of Power." For over two hours, women came forward in tears to confess sin and to pray in front of the assembled group! As the retreat ended on Sunday, many signed up for one day of a corporate forty-day fast that began the following day.

> *My only regret about my fasting is that I didn't start sooner. It grieves me when I look back on all the years that I settled for less than the best.*

My only regret about my forty days of prayer and fasting, as well as fasting a day a week these past two years, is that I didn't start sooner. It grieves me when I look back on all the years that I settled for less than the best. But these verses give me encouragement about the future: "Unless a kernel of wheat falls to the ground and dies, it remains only a single seed. But if it dies, it produces many seeds. The man who loves his life will lose it, while the man who hates his life in this world will keep it for eternal life. Whoever serves me must follow me; and where I am, my servant also will be. My Father will honor the one who serves me" (John 12:24–26).

৵

Student after student walked in with a Bible. It suddenly hit me—this was one of Jonathan Edwards' *Distinguishing Marks of a Work of the Spirit of God!* Edwards penned this classic work during the First Great Awakening (1741) to help people distinguish a genuine work of God from mere emotionalism. I retraced in my mind Edward's five distinguishing marks of a genuine work of God: 1. It raises the esteem of Jesus; 2. Satan's kingdom suffers as the Spirit of God strikes out against sin; 3. Men and women will have a greater respect for Scripture; 4. Men and women will see more clearly spiritual truth and error; 5. There will be a new sense of love toward God and others.

—John Avant, et al.
"Revival at Wheaton College," *Revival!*

Eddie and Alice Smith

The Smiths, who live in Houston, Texas, direct many intercessory prayer organizations, including U.S. Prayer Track and the Intercessory Prayer Network, Inc. They also publish a monthly prayer newsletter, Watchmen National Prayer Alert. *Alice has published several books on intercessory prayer, the most recent of which is* Beyond the Veil: God's Call to Intimate Intercession. *They serve as coordinators of* **PrayUSA!**, *a national prayer initiative. The Smiths have also begun a* First Friday *newsletter, which unites believers in fasting and prayer on the first Friday of every month to pray for specific needs in the Church and the nations.*[7]

Their work with **Pray USA!** *is calling Christians to prayer for revival in our country.*

I'm sure that no one needs to convince you that America is in desperate need of prayer. While we are seeing the worst corruption and immorality our nation has ever known, we are also seeing clear signs of revival on the horizon. It is time for us to discover what God is doing and partner with Him in it.

PrayUSA! is a national call to thirty days of prayer and fasting for revival and spiritual awakening. It is organized under the umbrella of the Mission America prayer initiative and chaired by Steve Bell of Concerts of Prayer International. The first meeting was held in April 1997 with more than one hundred leaders representing a diverse cross-section of our nation's prayer mobilizers (Concerts of Prayer International; Promise Keepers; March For Jesus, USA; Mission21–Houses of Prayer; AGLOW International; the Southern Baptist Convention; Denominational Prayer Leaders Network; and many more). The leaders have covenanted to mobilize prayer and fasting throughout the whole Church for revival and spiritual awakening in America. **PrayUSA!** provides neutral ground on which to rally all the U.S. prayer ministries so that they can compliment one another and facilitate revival.

Through **PrayUSA!**, Christians are offered an array of prayer possibilities, as well as a thirty-day prayer calendar/guide. They are also furnished with resource information. One focus is to mobilize intercessors to "pray on-site with insight" at one of thirty pre-selected "spiritual trouble sites." Teams of intercessors will travel to these sites, which are scattered across the United States, to fast, pray, and repent for past sins committed that may have given the enemy advantage (Nehemiah 1:4–11).

On the last Sunday of the thirty-day emphasis, pastors are encouraged to lead their churches in a "national day of repentance" or solemn assembly. **PrayUSA!** culminates with the National Day of Prayer (May 1) and March For Jesus (May 17).

⌇

The path toward humility is death to self. When self is dead, humility has been perfected (see Galatians 2:20). Jesus humbled Himself unto death, and by His example the way is opened for us to follow. A dead man or woman does not react to an offense. The truth is, if we become offended by the words of others, then death to self has not been finished. When we humble ourselves despite injustice and there is perfect peace of heart, then death to self is complete. Death is the seed, while humility is the ripened fruit.

—Alice Smith
Beyond the Veil: God's Call to Intimate Intercession

Wayne Atcheson

Wayne is the Sports Information Director for the University of Alabama. He shares how his fast started a chain of events in his personal life and in his work on the college campus that resulted in changed lives.

For the past eleven years, I have served as advisor of the Fellowship of Christian Athletes at the University of Alabama. In March 1995, I decided to begin my forty-day fast. I started in total faith and with much desire to have a challenging spiritual experience.

During my fast, I still played in charity and Christian golf events, carried on regular family activities, took my family out to eat, went to work everyday, worshipped as usual, and did my yard work and vacuuming.

On the twenty-second day, a very special blessing occurred. My college-age daughter needed minor surgery shortly after school ended. To make the long story short, the doctor [a personal friend] waived the $5,000 fee. He had no idea about my fasting. I did write him several weeks later about my fast and what a blessing he had been and how God had used him in our lives. I still reap the blessings of the forty-day fast and continue to fast each Wednesday.

Since that time, we have experienced some great changes during the Fellowship of Christian Athletes meetings. Shannon Brown is a 6' 5", 275-pound defensive tackle, a senior, and Alabama's top All-American candidate. The Sunday before school began, he had become so miserable that he decided to go to a church that he had never gone to before. At the invitation, he went forward and told the pastor, "I'm ashamed of the way my life is going. I can't go on this way. I need help."

The following Wednesday, he stood before our FCA group with tears and brokenness and expressed his new commitment before the athletes. Ten football players immediately surrounded him up front.

As I stood there watching this scene, I thought that if my fasting had anything to do with this, it was worth it all. When Shannon sat down, another big defensive tackle stood in the back and with tears shared how he had drifted from the Lord, too, but had decided to get right with the Him. Seventy-seven students were at that meeting. Word spread all over the athletic department. The next week, we had 154—twice as many. The following week, there were 200—more than ever in our thirty-two years of meetings.

On the Alabama campus this fall, our Christian groups and our church college assemblies have had more students attend meetings than ever before. The depth of our meetings has never been greater. We have had honest and open sharing as never before. We have had confession of sin, and many professions of faith. There has even been an expressed interest in fasting. We feel that revival is beginning to take place on our campus, for which we thank God.

ꜱ

> Clothe yourselves with humility toward one another, because, "God opposes the proud but gives grace to the humble." Humble yourselves, therefore, under God's mighty hand, that he may lift you up in due time. Cast all your anxiety on him because he cares for you.
>
> —1 Peter 5:5–7

Debra Clark

One of the most exciting aspects of the fasting and prayer movement is how Christians are bringing their convictions about fasting and prayer into areas in which they work. Debra Clark, who lives in Oklahoma City, shares her experiences in her career field as a physical therapist and with a related organization, Christian Physical Therapists International.

I'm a physical therapist, and I work with Christian Physical Therapists International. I'm the prayer coordinator for the organization. God laid it on my heart and my director's heart to begin fasting. Then God just continued to impress upon each of the board members to fast without our saying anything to each other. Eventually, all the board members spent time in fasting and prayer.

Two years ago, our board got together and in our human wisdom put down all these plans we felt we'd like to accomplish. We tried to accomplish them in our own strength and *nothing* happened. We started coming before Him in fasting and prayer, and now God has enabled us to complete all of those plans.

For example, we needed to get some publicity so people would have some way of knowing we existed. We wanted to take out an advertisement in our secular professional journal, but our budget was tight, so that didn't work out. Instead, someone contacted the head of our organization and did a phone interview with three of us. Not only were we publicized in our national magazine, but it ended up being a three-page insert! Then God opened the door for us to be in an *international* magazine for physical therapists. God gave us much more than we had imagined with hardly any effort on our part.

> *I've always had a call to prayer, but since adding fasting I've felt a different level of intensity and a sweetness in His presence.*

The publicity has resulted in additional membership and additional "arm raisers"—our prayer partners and financial supporters. We believe that this was a direct result of our fasting and prayer.

We also had a "*JESUS*" film outreach. We sent out free copies of the video to a certain group of our members. We know that three people were saved through the ministry of the video.

God has so impressed upon us that prayer is the issue that at our last board meeting, we put aside the agenda and prayed instead of doing a lot of planning.

I've always had a call to prayer, but since adding fasting I've felt a different level of intensity and a sweetness in His presence. I have a greater desire to be there. I also know that I don't fast so much for an answer, but for the sweetness of knowing Him. Usually, the answers come anyway.

ॐ

The Lord is good to those whose hope is in him, to
the one who seeks him; it is good to wait quietly
for the salvation of the Lord.

—Lamentations 3:25,26

International Fasting and Prayer

Political boundaries and national borders cannot stop God's work. I am confident that God is going to send a great spiritual awakening not only to our country, but also to the world. He is convicting His people —revealing their sin and the sins of their own countries— in preparation for a worldwide revival.

As this revival sweeps around the world, we will see renewed religious fervor. There will be a fresh awareness of the awesomeness of God and His attributes, a restoration of true worship, a hunger for the Word of God, and a new zeal to help fulfill the Great Commission and tell others the good news of God's love and forgiveness in our Lord Jesus Christ. We also will see a renewed vision for social issues and racial reconciliation.

Today, we see the beginnings of revival in many nations. For example, one of the most powerful movements of God in the world is in South Korea, where the Church is known as a praying Church. Its dynamic, dramatic growth from three million in 1974 to eleven million in 1990 can be attributed largely to fasting and prayer.

China has witnessed several remarkable revivals. Although missionaries have been barred from Mainland China since 1951, recent reports indicate that early missionary labors provided a base from which a vibrant, indigenous Chinese Church has developed. The Church in China, where fasting and prayer is commonplace, has grown from one million Christians in 1949 to nearly 100 million today.

And Latin America is in a sweeping revival! Researchers say that four hundred people are converted to Christianity in Latin America every hour. During the last decade, the Christian Church grew at a 220 percent increase, nine times the growth of the general population. No country in Latin America had gone untouched by spiritual revival.

To continue reaching the world that is so ripe for harvest will take commitment from the Body of Christ. I believe fasting and prayer are the keys to that commitment.

Now that you have read the testimonies from individuals and seen how God is working in churches, cities, and our nation, you can also begin to receive a vision for the world. As many Christians fast and pray for the parts of our world that the Lord lays on their hearts and then put their renewed faith into action, we will see the revival spread. I urge you to read the following testimonies with a prayerful attitude, asking God to give you a burden and a plan to link arms with others to reach the world for Christ.

Dick Eastman
Worldwide

Dick Eastman is president of the international ministry Every Home For Christ, and the author of over ten books on prayer. He lives in Colorado Springs, Colorado. His fast began as a personal journey, but expanded to include the leadership of his ministry.

I had felt for quite some time, leading into the month of October, that the Lord was guiding me into a forty-day fast. I direct the international ministry Every Home For Christ, which is in more than 110 countries with the goal of taking the gospel to every home in every nation. Our next goal is to begin campaigns to take the gospel to every dwelling in all the 1,739 unreached people groups that are defined by certain criteria. As we began to look at the challenge of reaching a minimum of a billion people, maybe more, who live in those areas, it just looked like the strategy presented a challenge far more complicated than we could possibly accomplish. I felt that, as the leader, I needed to spend forty days in fasting and prayer.

I had never before fasted for that long. October 19, 1996, represented the fiftieth anniversary of Every Home For Christ, which used to be known as World Literature Crusade. I thought it was appropriate to fast at the conclusion of our first fifty years and to look toward the amazing years ahead. As I was contemplating the decision to go ahead and try a forty-day fast, I knew there were many banquets coming up to celebrate our anniversary with key directors coming in from around the world. At first, I thought I would wait until January and start the new year. Then I heard that there were more than forty pastors and leaders in Colorado Springs who had decided to fast and pray beginning on October 8 and concluding on the final day of the Fasting & Prayer '96 conference in St. Louis. (Refer to the Colorado Springs citywide fast for details.) It was a confirmation to me that the Lord was indeed leading. I knew that with my type of schedule, there is no good time. I had all these celebrations, plus major meetings in London and regional directors meetings throughout my fast, but the Lord helped me.

One of the most significant things that has occurred in our ministry happened at the conference in St. Louis. I think it was first triggered by Nancy Leigh DeMoss.[8] I really began to think about how we plan. So often in ministry we do things the same way the world does, but just in a Christian context.

I came away from St. Louis with the idea that we should develop a whole new method of strategic planning in our ministry. I called it "Power Planning," a term that came to me as I was praying about it. At our bimonthly, two-day, strategic planning sessions, we now fast and pray. In strategic planning we usually deal with one issue and how to plan for it, then another issue. Previously, we would start the day in prayer, plan, then end in prayer. The Lord showed me that we needed to fast and keep our

Bibles open during our planning sessions. I've encouraged all of our executive team that at any time, any one of them can say, "I'd feel better if we'd pray over this." Periodically, we stop and pray over the last several issues discussed, then wait on God with open Bibles and listen to anything He says to confirm direction or to caution us.

We were dealing with some very difficult issues concerning our future, the ultimate goal of our ministry, and launching campaigns. There are so many directions to take, so many ideas of what we should do next, and the decisions are staggering. I just saw a clarity come through with this process, instead of confusion that can so easily happen when you're trying to work through something as challenging as reaching one billion people face to face— not via mass radio or television. We had to consider the logistics of going right to where they live, the translation of materials into their languages, and the strategies for reaching illiterate people.

When I completed my forty-day fast, a whole new passion seemed to seize me one day. I believe I'm filled with the Holy Spirit, but there was a passion for a far greater filling of the Holy Spirit in my life, to be much more controlled by the Holy Spirit. Samuel Chadwick, who wrote about being filled with the Holy Spirit, cited one of the indicators that he was filled with the Spirit: "God gave me a new Bible." I've always been daily in the Word and always have my prayer time, but the Bible just seemed like a brand new book to me. And in our meetings, I can sense among the group a whole new passion for the Word.

During the second week of the fast, I was with the group of ministers and leaders in Colorado Springs who were completing the forty-day fast together. One minister who works with juveniles in a youth detention center met with twelve very hardened teenagers who were in open rebellion. The center permitted him to share Jesus with them, and he said the results were unlike anything he had ever seen before.

"The presence of God came," the minister said, "and within a half-hour every single one of those boys bowed their head and received Christ as Savior. I have to believe that in some way fasting and prayer have caused this to happen."

The Lord has put upon us a fervent desire to do things His way and not man's way. We've seen spiritual warfare intensify dramatically in circumstances with the staff, as well as spiritual attacks on children where Satan seems to be trying to find a foothold in their lives. The battle is severe. The enemy is trying to rob us of the victory we have gained with the Lord. It's really important for people to complete these fasting seasons realizing that they have stirred up a "hornet's nest."

> *The Lord has put upon us a fervent desire to do things His way and not man's way.*

I think the Lord is reordering everything. We need a spirit of humility. One of the greatest problems in the ministry is that we are, in some ways, statistically driven. How many films do we have? How many countries are we in? How many workers do we have? How many salvation decisions? We think that next year we've got to do better, because if we don't have more to report, it will look like God is not blessing us. Pretty soon, we are actually driven by statistics and numbers. There can be a very subtle pride in our increased numbers.

I have felt that the Lord wants us to have a passion for the lost and rejoice in the results, but not get to the point where we are proud of the numbers. I think He's bringing us to a place of brokenness and humility before Him.

Over the years, everything I've written has been on prayer—more than ten books. I've developed a school of prayer that more than two million people have attended. I've spent many years trying to come to an understanding of what prayer is. Suddenly, I'm praying in new ways. Now

I find myself changing almost every one of my prayers, often with deep tears, "Lord, let us reach the lost *for Your name's sake.*" Everything is focused away from us and for the sake of His name throughout the world. It is a whole new burden that consumes me—*for His name's sake and glory*—not just to accomplish a task.

I feel that as we fasted and prayed together, many of the ministry leaders were knitted together in a deeper way. The group met every week. We had been discussing a joint building for over five years, but toward the end of the fast, there seemed to be a unified decision to go forward. There are very few cities of this size that have as many strategic ministries as Colorado Springs. So I really think God orchestrated this fast. A foundation of cooperation in working together has been established on a deeper level.

Until three years ago, I personally knew only two people in my entire life who had ever fasted for forty days. Now to think that hundreds and thousands are accepting this challenge amazes me. Fasting and prayer is becoming a foundation of almost everything we're doing.

꒜

Look carefully at some of our answers to prayer. Often, long before we ever thought to pray a particular petition, God set in motion certain events so that our prayer, when finally prayed, would be answered. Further, when examining some of these answers to our prayers, it becomes obvious that, even though God set in motion the answer before we actually prayed for a need, had we not prayed, certain circumstances could well have prevented our ever seeing the answer.

—Dick Eastman
The Jericho Hour

Phil Parshall
Philippines

Phil Parshall has been a missionary in Bangladesh and the Philippines for the past thirty-five years. His mission is to bring the gospel to Muslims.

For many years I have been deeply concerned about seeing our Lord give a breakthrough in the great task of Muslim evangelism...The question of "spiritual desperation" has haunted me. Have we paid the price of sustained prayer and fasting in order to bring about a significant turning to Christ from among the "sons of Ishmael"?

During this fast, I was able to walk, at least to some small measure, in the sandals of the poor and deprived. Instead of being able to eat anything I want at any time I want, I was able to suffer the hunger pangs, unfulfilled desires, and weaknesses of literally millions of the oppressed throughout the world. Also, thirty days of the fast took place during the month of Ramadan, so there was an identification with the Islamic world.

Thirteen Filipinos and missionaries kept the total forty-day fast. Perhaps twenty others fasted part of the time. A good number joined in around the world. I feel fulfilled in the vision the Lord gave me last September to promote this fast among those who minister to Muslims. And I am grateful to Bill Bright for his example, starting at age seventy-one, both in keeping the fast and in being the first to widely disseminate the call for Christians to engage in a forty-day period of focused prayer and fasting for world revival.

2>

"I know the plans I have for you," declares the Lord, "plans to prosper you and not to harm you, plans to give you hope and a future. Then you will call upon me and come and pray to me, and I will listen to you. You will seek me

and find me when you seek me with all your heart.
I will be found by you," declares the Lord.

—Jeremiah 29:11–14

Wesley Campbell
Worldwide

The tremendous efforts of Wesley Campbell must be acknowledged. Wesley's passion for revival is demonstrated in his worldwide call for 100,000 intercessors who will fast and pray for forty days. He is senior pastor at New Life Church, British Columbia, and travels extensively with the message of renewal through fasting and prayer. He is author of Welcoming a Visitation of the Holy Spirit. *He encourages people to read* The Coming Revival *before beginning an extended fast.*

"When I read Dr. Bright's book for the first time, I couldn't sleep," writes Wesley Campbell. "At 1:30 a.m., I struggled with the conviction that I, too, should observe a forty-day fast. By 2:15 a.m., I was convinced that I should fast and pray, and that I would not surely die. By 3:00 a.m., I felt led to call others to the same. By 4:00 a.m., my heart was racing with the excitement about thousands of Christians humbling themselves in fasting and lifting up their voices in prayer for forty days—crying out the Welsh revival prayer, 'Oh Lord, send your Spirit for Jesus Christ's sake.' Finally, at 4:30 a.m., I drifted off to sleep determined to call a fast through the forty days of Lent from February 12 to March 23, 1997 (Palm Sunday)."

Soon after this early morning conviction, Wesley continued to preach on revival, now with the added incentive of encouraging others to fast and pray. Everywhere he preaches in his home country of Canada and throughout the world, he invites Christians to spend time before the Lord (at least one week) asking whether He has called them to a forty-day fast.

"I am asking you to join with me and thousands of other believers from various nations around the world as we form a small army of 100,000 intercessors," writes Wesley Campbell. "We will be a portion of the two million believers that Dr. Bill Bright believes will be raised up to fast and call out for revival for forty days."

In addition to the fast beginning February 12, a strategy has now been launched in which the next two years (1997 through the end of 1998) will be sectioned into eighteen forty-day fasting segments. In this way, approximately every six weeks a new fast will begin that Christians can initiate or join either as a churchwide or citywide fast.

At this time, fasts are in progress in Spokane, Washington; Dallas, Texas; Bakersfield and Crestline, California; Memphis, Tennessee; Kansas City, Missouri; Arbroath, Scotland; and Kelowna, British Columbia. These group fasts are crossing denominational and ethnic lines, and changing cities in tremendous ways. Pastors and prayer leaders of these areas are asked to gather a group and call people to join them. During their fast, they are asked to hold nightly gatherings for prayer.

Rev. Campbell has also established an Internet Web site (www.revivalnow.com) to promote the call for 100,000 intercessors. The site provides resources and a place for dialog for those wishing to participate in a forty-day fast (E-mail address: prayer@revivalnow.com). He plans to post information from around the world on corporate fasts and contact names. "I'm getting responses from all over the world—Croatia, Wales, Scotland, England, Australia, Cambodia, Thailand, and Mexico."

"I'm not coordinating the extensive aspects of what every city will do," Campbell explains. "I'm sounding the call, describing a strategy, and modeling it. How all the different cities mobilize is up to them. The pastors are being very creative, and they are all inventing various strategies for their area." I look forward to hearing how God will use this corporate humbling, repentance, and seeking His face for His kingdom and glory.

For this is what the high and lofty One says—he
who lives forever, whose name is holy: "I live in a
high and holy place, but also with him who is contrite
and lowly in spirit, to revive the spirit of the lowly
and to revive the heart of the contrite."

—Isaiah 57:15

Internet Corporate Fast Worldwide

An Internet site was established by Teresa Seputis for those interested in participating in a corporate fast during the forty days from February 17 to March 28, 1997 (Good Friday). I encourage you to let my office know of other Internet corporate fasting efforts and their results. You can do so by calling (888) 327-8464.

After explaining the call to fasting and prayer, the site gives the following invitation: "If you are feeling led to fast and pray for revival, but your church is not sponsoring a corporate fast, please consider joining in the Internet Corporate Fast. You do not have to fast the entire forty days; you may fast any portion of it, as God leads. It is intended to be a place for us to build community, to encourage each other during the fast, to ask questions, to share what God speaks to us as we fast and pray, etc. This is a place to build up and encourage, not to criticize, not to tear down, not to attack. It will also be a place to debrief after the fast and share what God has done."

Teresa explains, "I fasted and prayed for three days to seek God's will on whether or not to do a long fast. He directed me not only to fast, but to start this E-mail list/ community and invite others to fast with me." Within five days of establishing the site, more than ninety people had signed up to participate in the fast.

A prayer calendar is also available with a theme and Scripture passage for each of the forty days to use as a guide. Some of the themes are: humility, His power in us; repentance; the Great Commission; praise and rejoicing;

contentment; and obedience. Other days focus on praying for your city, state, country, the government, the lost,
the poor and needy, and spiritual leaders.

The Internet certainly has the potential to bring together a vast community of Christians worldwide who can
share in their desire to seek God's face. The result of this
mass effort upon the nations will surely be to break the
strongholds of evil and transform God's people into
agents of love to reach the lost for His glory.

~

I dream of a new movement of Christians who immerse all
their activity—not just their worship and evangelism but
also their political analysis and cultural engagement—in all-
night prayer meetings. I dream of a movement that thinks
as it prays; that plans careful strategies as it surrenders to
the Spirit; that prays for both miraculous signs and wonders
and also effective social reform; that knows in its heart that
nothing important will happen unless the Spirit blows
through its plans; and also that God has no back-up plan
to use angels if we humans fail to do our part. A biblical
combination of prayer and action will change the world.

—Ronald J. Sider
Genuine Christianity

Paul J. Jannu
Hawaii and India

*Paul, whose mother interceded for him through fasting and
prayer, has in turn interceded for others through his own fast. He
has formed a chain encouraging Christians in Hawaii and
India to fast and pray. He is a pastor in Waipahu, Hawaii.*

During my fast, I spent time reading the Word and writing
down the revelations that God gave to me. I've read the
Bible fourteen times from cover to cover prior to that fast,
yet every verse was a new verse. It was a new book I was

reading; it was just jumping out alive. The living Word of God was coming through and it was marvelous! I was praising God for giving me the riches of His glory!

My dad was an ordained minister in the Methodist church in India. My grandfather was a first-generation Christian who had three wives and thirty-three children. He was a head of a small Hindu village, and the whole village became Christians. Now there are hundreds of fourth-generation Christians there. I was named after Paul in the Bible, and was raised in the church. As a child, I would memorize whole books of the Bible.

But I spent many, many years denying everything about God. I came to the United States and lived in Las Vegas, and spent my time gambling, drinking, and the whole lot. I won a lot of money at the tables. When I was on a winning streak, I would tip two or three thousand dollars to the dealer! Satan really wanted me to stay in that world. I went spiraling down and down. I felt like I had done everything and seen everything, so I attempted suicide many times. I'm sure it was through my mother's fasting and prayer that the Lord led me out of all that. I was nearly forty-five at that time. It has been twenty years since I started living for Christ and became a pastor.

During this fast, my prayer was to intercede for the leaders of the world and the church leaders that there would be revival and thirst for the Lord Jesus Christ. I now have about sixty people in Hawaii fasting one day a week. We have formed a chain. In India, there are also people fasting for revival.

I have started the Fasting & Prayer Chain International[9] where people can sign up to fast and pray at a certain time, and also to have their requests prayed for by others. Through this, I see India turning to the Lord in a miraculous way.

Revival Is Coming!

The Lord has taken hold of His church and has begun to shake it awake. The dust that has too long gathered has started to fall away.

Why do I believe revival has begun? The answer lies in the conditions I described in *The Coming Revival:*

> During revival, the Holy Spirit persuades believers of their true condition and their need to repent and return to their first love. He inspires His servants to speak His fresh messages to the Church. And He uses those whom He inspires to help convince other believers of their need to drop their worldly pursuits and seek after God with all their hearts.[1]

The life-changing accounts printed within these covers repeatedly give evidence of deep repentance, a fresh love for the Lord, speaking out in a vibrant way, and convincing others to follow Jesus in fasting and prayer and in action. When the Church once again becomes a vessel God can use, He will descend with power and revival.

When the Church breaks down barriers between the races and denominations, of formal and informal styles, of poor and rich, there will be revival! We are reading testimonies of churches and cities banding together like never before—Jewish and Arab believers coming together. Asians, African-Americans, Hispanics, Caucasians, and others saying, "We believe in one God and one faith in Christ Jesus. How then can we live as though the other one does not exist?" The charismatics and the non-charismatics are reaching out to each other; the liturgical to the non-liturgical; the suburban "super" church to the inner-city neighborhood hall. Of course, we're not saying that we should demolish the differences. We should aim to *utilize* the differences for the Body's greater good and see them as tools for God to use in this world.

These changes are a beginning, a first step. Even so, "Come, Lord Jesus!" Descend on us so that this generation is rocked out of complacency so that the whining of those who would say "What's the use?" will soon turn to shouts of "Here am I, Lord. Send me!"

In my travels I am seeing that the so-called Generation-X'ers on our college campuses are hungry for revival and are bursting with a fresh love for the Lord. Many have a great thirst for God and desire to follow Him. They are not willing to see the Church continue in a business-as-usual routine. The Holy Spirit is stirring up the youth of this country to force their church leaders to wake up and change.

The young—and not so young—are logging onto the Internet and finding others of like mind who want to fast and pray for revival when perhaps their own church isn't interested. They've found a new road to make this happen, and pretty soon their local churches will be stirred by God to sit up and listen.

Fasting with prayer is again becoming a priority for many, not just for the faithful few. Something is happening when the 1997 winning Superbowl football team kneels and prays to thank the Lord on the field! Thousands came every night for forty nights to experience God in Houston, Texas! A million Christian men will march in Washington, D.C., in October 1997 as part of Promise Keepers' "Stand in the Gap." Let us show this nation our love and resolve—and dissolve the image that they have of the Church as narrow, bigoted, uncaring, and condescending.

On the last day of my third forty-day fast, I was on my knees praying, "Lord, is there anything else you want to say to me before I end this fast?" I felt no impressions or unusual stirrings at that time. A few hours later, however, I was sitting in a Mission America meeting listening to reports about what God was doing across America:

- Southern Baptist churches working together in fasting and prayer

- Hundreds of denominations and groups setting aside one or two days a week to fast, pray, and seek God

- Tens of thousands of churches that are praying, fasting, and believing God for a new visitation of His presence

As the testimonies continued, the excitement and expectancy in that room crescendoed into praise and worship to our mighty and faithful God. Here I sat only one hour from my final prayer before breaking my forty-day fast, feeling and hearing nothing from God. Suddenly, His presence flooded my soul and I heard His gentle prompting, "Bill, what is happening in this meeting today is one of the greatest spiritual events of the centuries." The spirit of love, harmony, burden, and purpose rose with me that morning. I realized that this movement is unprecedented in this century, perhaps even in the history of the church. God is doing an amazing work throughout America and around the world just as He promises in Isaiah:

> I will pour water on the thirsty land, and streams on the dry ground; I will pour out my Spirit on your offspring, and my blessing on your descendants. They will spring up like grass in a meadow, like poplar trees by flowing streams (Isaiah 44:3,4).

My good friend Dr. Larry Lewis, former president of the Southern Baptist Convention Home Missions Board and now on staff with Mission America, tells the story about a young man who is a dedicated surfer. He surfs almost every day. One day Larry asked him why he did not go surfing that particular day. He quickly replied, "No waves." Dr. Lewis goes on to explain that we do not create spiritual waves, we just ride them. When God troubles the waters, when He stirs the current, when His Spirit is moving, we need to go out into the sea of our market places, get up on those boards of opportunity, and ride the waves to victory for the glory of God.

Have You Seen the Lord?

A forty-day fast before the Lord is a beginning. We learn, many of us for the first time, what it is to see our sin the way God does, to truly humble ourselves, and to seek Him with our whole heart, mind, and strength. Why does God have such strong emphasis on the importance of our confession, personal holiness, repentance, and a broken and contrite spirit?

Isaiah was a man after God's heart who had a burden to please the Lord. He was constantly calling attention to the sin of the people. Then something happened in his life:

> The year King Uzziah died I saw the Lord! He was sitting on a lofty throne, and the Temple was filled with his glory. Hovering above him were mighty, six-winged angels of fire. With two of their wings they covered their faces; with two others they covered their feet, and with two they flew. In a great antiphonal chorus they sang, "Holy, holy, holy is the Lord Almighty; the whole earth is filled with his glory." Such singing it was! It shook the Temple to its foundations, and suddenly the entire sanctuary was filled with smoke. Then I said, "My doom is sealed, for I am a foul-mouthed sinner, a member of a sinful, foul-mouthed race; and I have looked upon the King, the Lord of heaven's armies." Then one of the mighty angels flew over to the altar and with a pair of tongs picked out a burning coal. He touched my lips with it and said, "Now you are pronounced 'Not guilty' because this coal has touched your lips. Your sins are all forgiven" (Isaiah 6:1–7, TLB).

Isaiah said, "I saw the Lord!" And he was aware of his sin in new ways he had never even considered before. Have you seen the Lord? If there is pride in our life, or lust, dishonesty, anger, conflict, whatever it may be, God views it as sin. If we agree with God about our sin, we call the sin by name—confess it specifically. Repentance isn't saying, "Well, you know how I am, Lord." Confession is more than admitting, "A man has to do what he has to do!" If our attitude is properly changed, we will change our action. If there's no change in action, there is no true confession.

God is a just, holy, righteous God. He doesn't tolerate a superficial kind of Christianity. So I ask you, are you willing to step out in a new way for the Lord?

The Israelites were told over and over to dedicate themselves totally to the Lord. Aaron wore a small gold plate fastened to his turban emblazoned with the words *Holy to the Lord*. The word "holy" is often regarded in a negative tone today. It has come to be seen as thinking we are too good for others, self-righteous, off on a cloud somewhere, and not established in the real world. But that is not what the Bible means by being holy.

When God called His people to holiness, He was telling them to remember that we are a part of Him. We are set apart, marked for God, followers that cannot be turned to the left or the right. We are to be His fearless, love-filled, glorified Body on this earth.

Moses was commanded to make a holy oil with which to anoint Aaron and his sons as priests and to anoint the tabernacle so that all would be dedicated and consecrated to the Lord. In Exodus 30:29, we read, "You shall sanctify (separate) them, that they may be most holy; whoever and whatever touches them must be holy (set apart to God)" (Amplified). This oil was a symbol of the Holy Spirit.

Jesus quoted Isaiah: "The Spirit of the Lord is on me, because he has anointed me" (Luke 4:18). Hearing these words, the Jews knew immediately that Jesus was claiming to be the Messiah. Acts 10:37,38 says, "You know what has happened...how God anointed Jesus of Nazareth with the Holy Spirit and power, and how he went around doing good and healing all who were under the power of the devil, because God was with him." The anointing of Jesus marked Him as God's own.

We have been marked as God's own as well. In 2 Corinthians 1:21, Paul writes to believers, "It is God who makes both us and you stand firm in Christ. He anointed us, set his seal of ownership on us, and put his Spirit in our hearts as a deposit, guaranteeing what is to come."

Anointed, consecrated, dedicated—we have been made a part of the divine priesthood that calls us to walk with the living, ruling God of the universe. We can't live an anointed life apart from the Holy Spirit. We can't witness apart from the His power. Jesus said, "You will receive power when the Holy Spirit comes on you" (Acts 1:8). The Holy Spirit is the one who enables us to know the Lord Jesus. If we are willing to let God do what He wants to do in our hearts, and by faith claim the fullness of the Spirit of God, we will be spiritually robust, filled with His power to introduce others to Christ.

When we talk about an encounter with the living God, we must be sure that this encounter results in a dedicated life and a fruitful witness for Christ. The Holy Spirit is moving through us, guiding us, instructing us every day. When that happens, we thrive on studying the Word of God, learning the attributes of God, and trusting Him with every area of our lives. We readily confess our sins. We surrender our pride and our old self-seeking patterns for His ways and walk in humility.

The Lord does not want churches to remain hollow shells of feel-good fellowships. As believers, we are each responsible to live a holy life, to obey, to love God with all of our heart, soul, mind, and strength—to trust Him no matter what we see.

Power to Overcome Evil

We begin by humbling ourselves through fasting and prayer. If we fast and pray, it changes our sensitivity, our behavior, our thoughts, our relationships, our business plans, our leisure pursuits. If there is no change in our lives, quite honestly, fasting can be a waste of time.

In fasting, our Lord meets us and lifts up our heads and sets us on a higher path. For many of us, the forty-day fast was a mountaintop experience. Like Moses, we come down from the mountain and our faces glow with the glory of the Lord that we experienced. Every part of our lives seems to reveal the mysteries of God.

It is an amazing and wonderful experience that I pray each and every one of you can have. However, as we see from Jesus' fast, the end of the fast is the time when the evil one strikes. Satan will try to trip you up at your weakest point just so you doubt the brokenness and spiritual work accomplished through your extended fast. You may then see yourself as worse off than before the fast. Or you may see yourself as unworthy to be used of God.

We have to prepare for this attack. Just when you may be tempted to put up your spiritual feet to rest, you should put on your armor instead. Jesus warned His disciples, "Get up and pray so that you will not fall into temptation" (Luke 22:46). Temptation or persecution may come during your fast, two months later, or a year later. Satan wants you to feel as though you have failed in your walk with the Lord or that whatever you experienced during the fast was not real. Pray ahead of time and be prepared. If you stumble, remember that we are not condemned. Christ intercedes for us in all things. Confess and begin again. Do not be tempted to do a slow slide to mediocrity or hardness.

Pray also that you will not be tempted to think of yourself as "super spiritual" because you completed a forty-day fast. Let us never forget that if the Lord had not brought us through, we would not have made it nor experienced Him in our fasting. It would have been a mere work of the flesh. My prayer is that no one will even think that he is further along spiritually because he fasted more than someone else. The point is to *humble ourselves*—and stay humble!

Also, remember to share your new excitement and commitment for the Lord with others in love. In the Body of Christ, some Christians think that when people get on fire for the Lord, they need to burn down their church. In other words, they criticize the leadership, notice all the faults of the programs, and become impatient with others who are spiritually weak. This attitude only brings divisiveness. It is also the way Satan creeps in. Only the Holy Spirit can awaken the hearts of others. When we share our experiences of fasting and prayer in love and humility, others will want to fast and pray too. When they see our new life in Him, they will seek us out and desire to know more about a dedicated life. Bashing others over the head with "what needs to be done around here" won't change the church.

Pray for the church; love the church; serve in the church; lead by example. When you see problems, take them to God alone (not to others on your coffee break) for His provision. Open your eyes to the ways our Lord wants to change you in that circumstance. Pray that the church will be a golden reflection of Jesus Christ. Pray especially to love and encourage your pastor and church staff. They often carry a load that is beyond their abilities to bear. Let them know that you care by your actions as well as by your words.

I cannot say this too strongly: Earnestly pray for America. My close friend Chuck Colson describes America as a country in danger of losing its very soul. Ordinary, casual prayers will not overcome the evil in this land. No solution apart from the gospel of Jesus Christ and the mercy of

God will save us. Oh, how this nation needs serious fasting, prayer, and taking God at His Word.

Ask God for a vision for big things. Do you have a God-given vision for your life? For your family? Your church? Your community? Have you asked God to give you His vision for you and those in your world? Do you ask Him to reveal how you can reach people for Him through your influence?

Then after the forty days, stay close to the Lord. Follow Him and what He is doing.

When Will We See Revival?

Revival is a sovereign act of God, a divine visitation of His grace. Throughout history, revival has come in response to the Lord's stirring of His people. We cannot fast and "pray down" revival. We cannot repent and humble ourselves or serve hard enough to tip the balance of the scales to slide revival our way. God sent His only, dearly loved Son, Jesus Christ, to pay our great debt, and nothing else is needed or can satisfy our perfect, holy God. Our obedience, repentance, humbling, and serving is a response to what He has *already done*.

> *America [is] in danger of losing its very soul. Ordinary, casual prayers will not overcome the evil in this land.*

However, when we meet God's conditions, He will hear and answer us according to 1 John 5:14,15. God promised King Solomon that "if my people, who are called by my name, will humble themselves and pray and seek my face and turn from their wicked ways, then will I hear from heaven and will forgive their sin and will heal their land (2 Chronicles 7:14).

As human and imperfect fathers and mothers, we sacrifice to care for our children and meet their needs. We pay the price. Even in our imperfection, when our children ask for something special that we know would be good for them, we may wait for the right time to give it to them. We watch to see if they obey us and do the work we have asked them to do. We check on the way they treat their brothers and sisters. Sometimes we want them to ask us over a period of time so we are sure that their desires have not changed. We may foresee a good opportunity that the child cannot understand.

I can only assume this is how our heavenly Father regards our desire for revival. He is looking, checking, listening; He knows the best time. We cannot *earn* it, but we can demonstrate to our Father that we are ready, willing to do whatever it takes, fervently desiring revival.

Those who have experienced a touch of revival know its power. When it happens, the Holy Spirit takes over. Confession breaks out; people weep; meetings go on for many hours; and people are changed.

Alvin Reid, professor of evangelism at Southeastern Baptist Theological Seminary, co-authored the book *Revival!*, which retells what happened when revival came to a small church in Brownwood, Texas, and spread across the country. He had studied revivals for many years and knew what to do when suddenly one Sunday revival came and nothing was the same. Reid says, "As Americans, we're control freaks—and we haven't prepared pastors for this eventuality. The Spirit can move in disorganized ways, but that doesn't mean chaos. A service can go on for three or four hours, you may have unusual confession of sin, but it doesn't have to be chaos."[2]

Reid recommends that churches keep the revival spirit alive, without chaos, by using the following guidelines:

1. Guard against extremism or the latest fads of "charismania."
2. Confess private sin *privately*, especially sins that involve other people.

3. Be kind to church members suspicious of revival.

4. Keep the focus on Bible teaching, not emotion.

5. Don't exaggerate what's happening; don't become too proud.[3]

Revival will come when God deems it is best for His purposes. Until then, we follow His Word, we humble ourselves, and we work to fulfill the Great Commission.

Prepare for the Harvest

When revival comes and when believers repent and follow the Lord in a revolutionary way, the supernatural love of God will be manifested in their personal lives and in all of their relationships. Renewed Christians will seek to be world-changers in schools, government, and business, as well as in the church. They do not have to resort to the world's evil ways of accomplishing change. They will be grieved and turn away from anything that makes light of lust, violence, and a godless society. Revolutionary believers will use the supernatural love of Christ to attractively change the way the media and individuals regard the Church. By loving their neighbors, praying for and blessing their cities, working for the good of Christ's kingdom, and supporting Christian outreach endeavors (missions, the poor, widows, orphans, prisoners, and others), the people of the world will see God and want to know Him for themselves.

The challenge for world evangelization is great. To accomplish the task, God will empower and work through His children who totally surrender themselves to His will. He works supernaturally through yielded, Spirit-filled followers.

When God sends revival, hundreds of millions will come into the kingdom. With all the resources available to us, we are the most privileged of all the Christians throughout the centuries. As we end this second millennium and launch into the third, we have the manpower, the money, the technology, the strategies, and everything we need to complete the task of fulfilling the Great Commission.

I am personally persuaded that from 1980 through the end of 2000 A.D., there will be over one billion new believers. They need to be followed up, discipled, and trained in their new faith. In turn, they need to understand the concept of sharing that faith with many others,[4] which Paul gives in 2 Timothy 2:2. I am not surprised at what God is doing in these last days. It is just a prelude to what we will see happen by the end of the century.

> *What God is doing in these last days.. is just a prelude to what we will see happen by the end of the century.*

At Campus Crusade for Christ, we are anticipating and preparing for huge numbers of new believers by offering discipleship training. With the technology now available to us, we are preparing to train tens of millions of people in at least 10,000 New Life Training Centers. We will also train through seminars, radio, books and study guides, the Internet, CD ROM, interactive learning, and all the other instruments God has made available to us.

Still, what good is the technology without Christians willing to not only evangelize, but also build up these new believers? Prayerfully consider God's call on your life to love and serve our Lord and His Church in this way.

To the church leaders, I want to give an "early warning" message. Many will recall that in the early 1970s a revival of the Jesus movement or "Jesus People" flourished for a short time amid the draft card burnings, anti-war rallies, riots, and LSD use that marked those years. Often when these new "hippie" converts entered established churches, they were met with disdain for their long hair and tie-dyed clothing. Some decided to conform and were accepted by traditional churches. Others started their own churches where they could worship Jesus in bell-bottom jeans, platform shoes, and long hair. Unfortunately, many left the church, which they saw to be hypocritical and not having the love of Jesus that first drew them to our Lord.

Now we are at the end of the twentieth century. Young people often like to dress in unusual clothing (oversized, skimpy, or outrageous). Many have tattoos, various body piercings, shaved heads, or brightly colored hair. These young people have derived much of their theology from MTV and TV situation comedies, which teach them that life is about being provocative, greedy, and self-centered. When Jesus Christ reaches out and brings them to Himself, He accepts them—but will we as the Church turn them away? Will they find a hymnal to share with a regular attender, or will we again close the door on those whom Christ wants to bring in?

I would like to challenge churches everywhere to go out and reach those young people—just the way they are! They will have a tremendous impact on the course of this country and the world in the twenty-first century. Love them no matter how they act or what they wear on Sunday morning, and they will see God in us. If we turn from them, we leave them to a life of drugs, promiscuity, despair, and perhaps an eternity in hell.

Let us beware of a spiritual arrogance that blocks out anyone who doesn't look or act the way we do. We must remember God's counsel to Samuel: "The Lord does not look at the things man looks at. Man looks at the outward appearance, but the Lord looks at the heart" (1 Samuel 16:7). Love in Jesus' name does not force others into our own agenda. Are we willing to give up our comfort zone? Drop our religious jargon? Get out on the front-lines? Open ourselves to other ways of doing things?

The key is being in love with Christ and really believing that we can love people into the kingdom through the enabling of the Holy Spirit. Fasting humbles us and enhances our intimacy and trust in our Lord and King. It returns us to our first love so that we can love God and others deeply. We never compromise the message of salvation and His holy Word. No matter what happens as a result of fasting, prayer, and the moving of God's Spirit, let Christ be the judge of all things. We, on the other hand, must remain faithful to loving, obeying, serving, praising, and doing whatever He has called us to do for Him.

Where Do We Go From Here?

I received a letter from a businessman and educator with a successful fifty-five-year track record. He said that at an age when most people are in heaven or hell, retired or otherwise occupied in mundane affairs, he is starting a new business that will have worldwide impact for the kingdom of God. Yes, at eighty years of age, he wants to make a difference.

God is doing so many dramatic, revolutionary things through Campus Crusade for Christ and other ministries. It is my prayer that God will speak to you and call you to be a part of this movement to help change the world through helping fulfill the Great Commission—the greatest challenge ever given by the greatest Person who ever lived.

God has revealed hundreds of projects, ministries, and other key ways to accelerate the spread of His message throughout the nations of the world. As of January 1, 1997, He had brought more than 14,200 full-time staff and 163,000 trained volunteers in 167 countries to Campus Crusade for Christ to help us. Our staff is partnering with about 500 mission groups and agencies throughout the world. God has blessed the faithful efforts as literally millions of people worldwide have indicated that they have received Jesus Christ as their Savior and Lord. Vonette, my dear companion and co-laborer, and I know in our hearts that we have accomplished nothing apart from God—that every positive result of our labors is only because of His blessing and supernatural work in the hearts of people. We are only His instruments, trying to remain faithful to His calling. If we should ever make the prideful mistake of thinking we can do it by ourselves, He could quickly remove His hand of blessing from us. God uses the humble, broken, obedient, and surrendered heart, not the proud, boastful one. Therefore, we know that now more than ever, we must be on our knees before Him in a spirit of confession, humility, and obedience to His will.

My burden is to go forth with the guidance and enabling of the Holy Spirit, to continue and improve our existing ministries worldwide, and to develop and implement exciting new strategies designed to "step up the pace" toward ushering in true revival upon our families and churches. Working hand-in-hand as teammates with other Christian organizations, denominations, and independent churches, we are dedicated to using the most strategic, efficient means available to give every resident of Planet Earth the opportunity to say "yes" to Jesus Christ. There simply is nothing more important for Christians to be doing.

You may ask, "What does all this have to do with me?"

Let me encourage you to determine just how He wants to make your life count the most for eternity. Will you join us in faithfully fasting, praying, and believing that God will continue to bless and use us—even in greater ways than in the past? Will you help us pray for one million godly, Spirit-filled, qualified Christian men and women to join us as full-time or part-time associates and trained volunteers in the task of saturating the world with God's message of love and forgiveness? Will you consider being part of the number needed to accomplish the new vision and strategies the Lord has given to us?

I am also asking the Lord to lay on the hearts of two million people to join me in forty days of fasting and prayer for revival. Will you be one?

Finally, I want to ask those of you who have completed an extended fast in which God has done something special to share with others your experiences with fasting and prayer. When you write your testimony of the impressions, inspirations, challenges, or results you experienced, you will greatly encourage and bless others to seek God in this way. The Response Form at the end of this book will provide further instructions on how you can send your testimony to me.

The fields are ripe unto harvest. There is growing evidence that revival fires are starting to burn across America and around the world. Millions of people are realizing the futility of life apart from God and are turning from their wicked ways. More hearts and doors are open now than ever before in history. As we humble ourselves before God and obey His command to share Christ in the power of the Holy Spirit, revival fires will burn brighter and brighter in the days ahead. The world is primed and ready for the Good News of Jesus Christ, but as Paul asked, "How can they believe in him if they have never heard about him? And how can they hear about him unless someone tells them?" (Romans 10:14, TLB).

There is no nobler calling, no better investment of one's life than telling others how to know God personally and enjoy Him forever.

Revival is coming! In fact, sparks of revival are igniting all over this nation and throughout the world. The fruits and blessings of revival are ready for the taking. As we participate in this fasting and prayer movement of God, we look forward to being part of this revival. We want you to be part of it, too! Will you join us in this exciting adventure? Will you join us in fasting, praying, believing, giving, and going?

Will you come help us change the world?

Call to Prayer

By Bishop Carlton D. Pearson

I'm elated to be here this morning. This is the third event of this type that Dr. Bill Bright has been led to initiate and orchestrate with his wonderful staff. It's my second time being here, and I feel so honored to be in the presence of praying people—fasting and praying people.

I will talk to you from Romans 8:22, "We know that the whole creation has been groaning as in the pains of child-birth." That means a lot to me because my wife had a baby two weeks ago, our second little child, and I was in the room. I was groaning with her, and it was like a prayer. Notice how Paul mixed the metaphor: "We know that the whole creation has been groaning as in the pains of child-birth right up to the present time. Not only so, but we ourselves, who have the firstfruits of the Spirit, [sigh or] groan inwardly as we wait eagerly." That word, *wait*, in the Greek actually means to watch with outstretched hands, constrained expectation, eager longing. "We wait eagerly for our adoption as sons, the redemption of our bodies. For in this hope we were saved" (vv. 22–24). The King James Version says, "We are saved by hope: but hope that is seen is not hope: for what a man seeth, why doth he yet hope for?"

Bishop Pearson is Senior Pastor of Higher Dimensions Family Church in Tulsa, Oklahoma; and Founder, President, and Presiding Bishop of Azusa Interdenominational Fellowship of Christian Churches and Ministries. This address was presented at Fasting & Prayer '96 in St. Louis, Missouri, November 15, 1996.

One interesting thing about prayer, one of the ingredients of prayer is waiting. Another ingredient is hoping, and still another is groaning. He goes on to say in verse 26, "In the same way, the Spirit helps us in our weakness. We do not know what we ought to pray." There's another word for prayer in Greek that means to wrap yourself around God and to beg, almost to plead with Him, for certain recognition. Here, he's saying the word most commonly used for prayer in the New Testament: to want, to wish, or to desire; to need, sometimes used to mean to worship. Paul is saying that we don't know how to worship.

The reason many people don't pray is because they don't know how to pray. Paul says we don't know what to want; we don't know what to need or desire or what is required. The Holy Spirit makes intercession for us. He actually intervenes. He actually goes in the inner sanctum of the presence of God and discerns the mind of God, gets the intention of God, and prays for the saints—not according to their prayers—but according to the will of God. The Holy Spirit not only intercedes, but He sometimes interrupts or intervenes or intercepts. Sometimes, He actually interferes because we don't know how to pray as we ought. As we pray, the Holy Spirit will actually intercept that which is not necessarily in the will of God, not in connection with the divine, and He takes our prayers right into the presence of God, and those are the prayers that are answered. "He who searches our hearts." That means, He who investigates or inquires of our hearts—knows the mind and the intentions and purposes—prays for the saint according to the will of God. And the next verse says, "And we know that all things work together."

After forty-three years of living on the planet, I have never wanted God like I want Him now. Our being here doesn't say that we are super-religious or super-spiritual. It says that we want God, we're desirous of God. We want to breathe God and know God and worship God. That happens in prayer and also in our fasting. The word for fasting literally means "to cover the mouth." Really, it means to cover the entrances or accesses to the innermost being. Sin came into this world through our mouths—eating. The devil likes to interrupt our eating. There will be a final wedding supper of the Lord. Feasting and fasting have a lot to do with the Christian discipline, with the walk of the believer. To cover the entrances also means to sometimes cover the eyes or the ears from what you take into your spiritual system.

> *The word for fasting literally means "to cover the mouth." Sin came into this world through our mouths—eating.*

My mother used to tell me that praying and fasting were two wings of the same bird. My parents had us fasting when I was only twelve years old. They would go seven days, fourteen days, twenty-one days, and they would make us children fast until noon. Mother made us stand around her while she prayed. I remember that. Over the years, I've learned the discipline of fasting and praying. Those times, I just simply wanted God.

I was birthing something. I'm telling you, folks, you are going to leave here pregnant. You actually came here pregnant, and your prayer is part of the birthing process. You are being "midwifed" by the Holy Spirit.

Rather than a doctor this time, my wife and I used a midwife. We were pushing and there were groanings and mutterings. When the baby crowned, the midwife said, "Okay, Papa, take over." With my fingers right on my little girl's face, I just gave a very gentle pull and out she popped! And I burst into tears! I quickly clipped the umbilical cord and lifted her straight up to God and said, "Father, I give her back to you just like You gave her to me. I'm persuaded that He is able to keep that which I've committed unto Him."

Whatever you're praying, you are committing unto God, and God's going to honor it. He says in Jeremiah, "Call for the wailing women." That means those who know how to birth, those who know how to travail and groan and want this child, want this event to take place—whether it's your marriage or business or ministry or nation. We are birthing something in America, right here in St. Louis. The Body of Christ has come together cross-denominationally, cross-culturally, and we are birthing something in the Holy Spirit that's going to affect this nation and take us into the twenty-first century as a victorious church and a delivered nation.

Finally, Isaiah 66:9 says, "'Do I bring to the moment of birth and not give delivery?' says the Lord." Proverbs says, "The seed of the righteous shall be delivered" (Proverbs 11:21, KJV). Let me make you a promise. Whatever you pray for, whatever you are "pregnant with in the Spirit," you are going to see it give birth. Your praying and your fasting are going to solemnly put us into another supernatural vein.

Let's enter a time of just seeking the Lord. I'm going to ask you not to ask for specifics right now, for He already knows what we need before we speak it. Prayer is just an act of faith. I want us to breathe deeply and just *want God.* Breathe God and emote God. Say, "God, I want You so much. I want to know You. I desire You. You are everything that I need and I want. I seek You with my whole heart."

Father, we thank You and we bless You and we honor You. You said, "Blessed are those who hunger and thirst for righteousness, for they will be filled" (Matthew 5:6). So right now, we hunger and we thirst. We've come from all across this continent and from even other parts of the world to collectively want You, to collectively need You, to collectively desire You. You said, if Your people who are called by Your name would humble themselves and pray and seek Your face and turn from our wicked ways, then would You hear our prayers; then would You hear from heaven, and will forgive our sin, and heal our land.

From the White House to the court house to the school house to the crack house to the dog house, we pray that the mighty manifestation of the supernatural power of God will deliver this nation. We are pregnant at the end of century and at the close of this millennium. Thank You that You have birthed faith in the heart of people. We seek You now. We ask for Your guidance.

We want You for our families. We want You for our marriages. We want You for our nation. We worship You in spirit and in truth. We don't even know what to want, but thank You, Holy Spirit, for quickening our hearts with the intelligence of heaven, clarifying our will. We submit to You our lives, our whole soul, mind, and body. We give You praise and we give You glory.

How Is God Calling You to Return to Him?

By Dr. Ronnie W. Floyd

God used fasting and prayer to bring a major change in my life. In fact, I could even go so far as to tell you tonight that it was through the ministry of fasting and prayer that God recently changed, not only my life, but also my ministry. Fasting and prayer brings death to self. And the more death to self we experience, the more we encounter the living Christ. When we begin to encounter the living Christ, we begin to understand more than ever before about the holiness of God. As we understand the holiness of God, we join with Isaiah in confessing to the Lord God how wicked and sinful we are.

My friends, tonight I want to challenge you with this thought: The more we learn to look up, the more we learn to look in and see our sinfulness before God. When we humble ourselves before God, which I believe comes only through fasting and prayer, we will enter into what I call God's gateway to supernatural power. Wouldn't you like to know the entry point into the supernatural power of God? Some of us might struggle when we hear that

Dr. Floyd is Pastor of First Baptist Church, Springdale, Arkansas, and Founder/President of Awaken America. He is also Chairman of the Executive Committee and President of the 1997 Pastors' Conference of the Southern Baptist Convention. This is condensed from an address presented at Fasting & Prayer '96 in St. Louis, Missouri, November 14, 1996.

word *supernatural,* but I want to remind you that if you know Christ as your Lord and Savior, it took a supernatural work by the Spirit of God. There is nothing to fear about the supernatural power of God. It simply means "above the natural." We need a lot of "above the natural" to go against our popular culture today.

Tonight, each one of us must understand this truth: We are losing America! Our nation is on a spiritual and moral slide that Satan has greased to lead this country to destruction. We are already under the mighty judgment of God. Consider the rampant sins of homosexuality, abortion, pleasure, greed, and idolatry that exist in this country. We are in great need for God to move in our midst. For too long America has seen what we can do in the church. In our own strength we have produced divided, mediocre, visionless, and powerless churches. It is time that America sees what God can do in and through the Church of Jesus Christ. I believe that God wants to show America His mighty power. This powerful God who raised Jesus from the dead lives within us and provides the power for effective living.

> *For too long America has seen what we can do in the church. In our own strength we have produced divided, mediocre, visionless, and powerless churches. It is time that America sees what God can do in and through the Church of Jesus Christ.*

Look at the churches of this country. We see the sin of unbelief in most of our churches. We see the sin of religious tradition in the church. The sins of pride, fleshly desires, and broken relationships abound everywhere. We need new wineskins for this day. Our old wineskins are lifeless and brittle; we need a new touch from the living

God. We are needy people—needy for a mighty move of the glory and the power of God.

God wants to release His supernatural power. What for? To awaken the Church. To empower believers to touch this country for Jesus and to take the gospel of Christ throughout the entire world. I know that this a very large task—an impossible task. And that is why we must get the God of heaven involved in our lives and ministries.

How do we do that? We reach for one of the greatest, most powerful weapons that the Church has at its disposal —the ministry of fasting and prayer.

What is fasting? Fasting is abstaining from food with a spiritual goal in mind. Fasting is neglecting the most natural desire of your body, which is for food, in order to appeal to the God of heaven to do something supernatural in your life, your ministry, or your nation.

I am reminded of what God taught me about fasting. No one ever taught me how to fast and pray. I grew up in a Baptist church not hearing much about fasting. When I was a freshman at a Baptist college in Texas, I had a strong desire to be all that God wanted me to be. One day when reading the Scripture, I began to learn what it meant to pray and fast. Who taught me how to fast and pray? The Holy Spirit of God. As I began to learn that truth and practice that discipline, I began to see God do some great things in my life and ministry.

On January 15, 1990, God began to do something new in my life, taking me to a new level. On that day, my thirty-five-year-old wife was diagnosed with cancer. For the next year, we did not know what her future held. We struggled through a hard year of surgeries, six weeks of radiation, and six months of horrible chemotherapy. I felt impressed that God wanted me to fast and pray one day a week for my wife's healing. And I can tell you tonight that since that time, the God of heaven has brought physical healing to my wife. To God be the glory!

God has since burdened me with the ministry of fasting and prayer. In 1991 I began to fast forty days a year, one day a week for forty weeks. During these days, I asked God for three or four things that He wanted me to trust Him for in those times of fasting and prayer.

Early one morning in March 1995, as I lay before the Lord in the basement of my home, the Spirit of God came into my heart on that morning and said, "Ronnie, I want you to fast and pray for forty days in a row that this nation might have spiritual revival, that your church might have spiritual revival, and that you might have and experience spiritual revival in your life."

At that time I was not aware of what had happened with Dr. Bright's fasting experience, nor of his book *The Coming Revival*. But it was probably his prayer that God had answered, because I was one of those people who didn't know anything that was going on about fasting for revival. Those forty days changed my life. All I can tell you is that I have never been the same since those days.

God grabbed my attention zeroing in on America, my church, and upon the sins in my life. One Saturday night as I prayed before retiring, I made what for me was a bold statement: "God, I am going to interpret all sleeplessness as a call to prayer." In the early morning hours, I found myself awake and sliding out of bed to pray. All of a sudden, the Spirit of God breathed a word from heaven to me out of Isaiah 57:15 and said to me, "Ronnie, the biggest problem in your church, the biggest problem in your ministry, and the biggest problem in your life is your pride—your sin of pride." And in a way that God only can tell you, He said, "Ronnie, you are a young, you are an arrogant, you are a proud pastor, and I am going to break you so that I can make you to be what I want you to be."

In those morning hours I felt like I had been taken to the woodshed. Those were hours when God came all over me with Holy Spirit conviction and touched my heart.

And when I got up that morning, I knew that I was free! Like never before in my life—free!

Friends, God wants to begin with you this week. He cannot begin with the nation and He cannot begin with the Church. A move of God begins with us. We are the problem. Yes, revival is determined by the sovereignty of God, but it is also determined by the condition of our hearts.

After my experience when God convicted and broke me over my pride, I felt impressed to tell my church people about it. On Sunday morning, June 4, 1995, I stood before my church and told them about the journey that God had taken me on for my forty-day fast. In the middle of my message, I told the people, "Listen, God is here today in an unusual way. You sit back and don't worry about the later Sunday school. We're going to go with it as long as God wants us to." Then God came in fresh power and anointing on the First Baptist Church of Springdale, Arkansas. He so interrupted that service, as well as the entire schedule of the morning, that the morning worship service went two-and-a-half hours. And people were on their faces before God in repentance over their own sin. Brokenness overwhelmed us. Worship and praise broke out all around us. When God shows up and helps you deal with your sin and hardness, you suddenly discover that in Him you're cleansed, free, and victorious. And your heart is filled with worship, praise, singing, and sharing.

I wondered if anyone would show up for the evening service that Sunday. To my surprise, seventy percent of that morning crowd came back that night. The service that night lasted over four hours with brokenness and confession of sin like I have never seen in my life. I learned something as a pastor that night. We have people in our churches whom we are asking to do a job in the Church for the kingdom, but they cannot do it because they are so bound in their sin. And the great news is that we have the release—the power of God that comes through the ministry of fasting, prayer, confession, and brokenness.

Without my calling any of my people to a forty-day fast, about fifty of our lay people have completed forty days of fasting and prayer. And many of their lives have been revolutionized by the power of God.

In January 1996, I was attending the clergy conference of Promise Keepers in Atlanta. While there, I kept praying, "God, would you please take our church to a new level? We need to know where you want us to go. I want to go all the way with You, Lord."

And God said to me, "Ronnie, if you want your church to go to a new level, you must first rise to a new level." In that dome stadium in Atlanta, the Holy Spirit of God called me to another forty-day fast. I believe this call to fasting was preparation for a wonderful opportunity that summer to deliver the Convention Sermon at the Southern Baptist Convention, one of two main addresses for the delegates from more than forty thousand churches.

On the twenty-second day of that fast, God gave me a word out of the Book of Joel. A strong word. A tough word. A word quite honestly that I was fearful of giving because I was afraid of the response by those pastors and church delegates attending the convention. I struggled that morning with obedience to God, but I knew God wanted me to do it. Once again God reaffirmed to me that if we will obey Him, He will take care of all things. And that morning I preached and offered the challenges that I believe God wanted given—that our denomination from October 27 to November 3 would simultaneously participate in calling our people to a sacred or solemn assembly. On October 27, 1996, in the morning church service, our pastors would preach on the subject of fasting, calling their people to observe October 30 as a day of humiliation, prayer, and fasting. In the evening service, we would lead our churches in a solemn assembly, a time when we cry out to God over our sins and the sins of our nation, begging for the mercy of God to come upon us. On November 3 we would preach in the morning and evening church services on the subject of spiritual revival, calling the people to it regardless of the cost, and asking God for His power to come upon the Church of Jesus Christ in America.

When the invitation was given that morning in our church, God moved in such a powerful way. It was unusual. You've seen it, I trust. It was a time when no one can explain what is happening, but you know that God touches the hearts of people. And many of our Southern Baptist churches by the thousands completed those special times with the Lord.

> *America is where it is because the Church is sick. The Church needs healing. And when the Church gets healed, America will become healed.*

Can I tell you about what happened in our church that first Sunday night? Solemn assemblies were not new to our church. But this time God began to move. We began to confess our sins and those of this nation.

America is where it is because the Church is sick. The Church needs healing. And when the Church gets healed, America will become healed. So the Holy Ghost of God came into that room, and, quite honestly, I've never seen such Holy Spirit conviction and brokenness. The only comfortable place in that building was on your face before God. It shouldn't have surprised me because earlier that morning more than sixteen hundred of our people signed commitment cards, walked down to the front of our church, laid them on the altar, and said, "Yes, on October 30, I will fast and pray all day long for revival in America." God honored the prayer and fasting of His people. God is doing some great things across this country.

Fasting and prayer is God's gateway to supernatural power. It places you in line to the supernatural power of God that many of you have never experienced in your life. So let me ask you tonight, do you desire God to do something supernatural in your life? In your ministry? Or in your nation? And let me take it to another level tonight. Are you desperate for God to do something in your life? In your ministry? Or in your nation? You've come to the right place to do business with God.

Some time ago, God spoke to me in the Book of Joel in a significant way. Would you look with me to Joel, chapter 2? The Bible says, beginning in verse 12: "'Even now,' declares the Lord, 'return to me with all your heart, with fasting and weeping and mourning.' Rend your heart and not your garments. Return to the Lord your God."

Oh, my friend, let me tell you tonight, God is calling us to return to Him. Note how God is calling us to return to Him—in prayer, in fasting, in weeping, in mourning. These are the conditions God has given us for coming to Him.

Then the Lord spoke to me about Joel 2:28–32. He said, "Ronnie, if you'll go on with Me, I'll fulfill Joel 2:28–32. Any Christian or church in America that wants to go on with God, I'll fulfill them in their midst." These verses say, "And it will come about after this." After what, ladies and gentlemen? After you have prayed. After you have wept. After you have mourned. After you have called a solemn assembly. After you have fasted. It will come about "after these things that I will pour out My Spirit on all mankind." That began to be fulfilled at Pentecost, but the autumn of fulfillment of that promise will take place just prior to the coming of Jesus Christ.

The Bible goes on to say,

> "Your sons and your daughters will prophesy, your
> old men will dream dreams, your young men will see
> visions. And even on the male and female servants I

will pour out My Spirit in those days. And I will display wonders in the sky and on the earth, blood, fire, and columns of smoke. The sun will be turned into darkness, and the moon into blood, before the great and awesome day of the Lord comes. And it will come about that whoever calls on the name of the Lord will be delivered" (NASB).

They will be saved. Do you believe that tonight? As you walk in and out of this place over the next few days, walk claiming, believing, and anticipating Joel 2:28–32 for this nation.

I close with this: How is God calling you to return to Him tonight? I challenge you in these next several minutes to get before God, whether it be on your knees, or just sitting or standing with Him. And ask the Lord these questions: "How are You calling me to return to You tonight?" "Am I willing to pay the price?" The destiny of millions of lost people in this country will be determined by our decision to obey God. Jesus is coming. We must pay the price. Come on back, come home to God right now.

Commitment
to Leaders

By Mrs. James C. (Shirley) Dobson

During the 1988 Summer Olympics in Los Angeles, the eyes of our nation's young people were focused on the medal-winning performance of our gymnast team. Afterwards, it came as no surprise that literally thousands of young Americans aspired to become gymnasts—it had been modeled for them on television.

Likewise, we look to our president as a role model; he is expected to be the spiritual and moral leader of the nation. Unfortunately, I think that some of the blame for the public's discontent with our government falls on *our* shoulders because we have not been praying for our leaders. First Timothy 2:1,2 says that we are to pray "for kings and all those in authority, that we may live peaceful and quiet lives in all godliness and holiness," in order that they may come to know the truth.

My husband, Jim,[1] and I are in leadership roles, although they are not political in nature. It is not easy being in that position. It creates special stresses on your marriage. There are unique dangers that sometimes befall your children. When my husband was appointed to the Attorney General's Commission on Pornography, we felt we were under attack by the Enemy. Our daughter was in

Mrs. Dobson is Chairman of the National Day of Prayer Task Force. This address was presented at Fasting & Prayer '96 in St. Louis, Missouri, November 15, 1996.

a car accident, and our son narrowly escaped being run over by a car. I told Jim, "When we get to heaven someday, and the curtain is pulled back, we are going to be amazed by all the pain our family and our ministry have been spared as a result of the faithful prayers of God's people."

The Scripture says, "Blessed is the nation whose God is the Lord" (Psalm 33:12). Unfortunately, we have people in leadership all across the nation whose God is *not* the Lord. We know that some of them are praying, but we don't know to *whom* they are praying, and we don't know *what* they are praying. I don't think they're praying to the living God.

> *As people of faith, we need to be on our knees praying for [our] leaders. They are making decisions that not only affect our lives but those of our children as well.*

As people of faith, we need to be on our knees praying for these leaders. They are making decisions that not only affect our lives but those of our children as well. In the National Day of Prayer Task Force office, we have initiated a project that we're calling "Adopt a Leader." All too often we have criticized our leaders but have not spent enough time interceding for them. We are asking people of faith to commit one year to adopting an elected leader and praying for them, if not on a daily basis, at least regularly. We are asking them to contact that leader's office once a month—not to be a pest, but just to say to them, "I want to encourage you. I want you to know I'm praying for you. I'm praying for your children. I'm praying for your wife or husband. I'm praying for God's protection around you. I know there is a piece of legislation coming across your desk—I'm going to be praying about that."

Please join us in taking on this challenge. We have an "Adopt a Leader" kit that we make available to churches, organizations, Sunday School classes, families, and individuals that will help you in praying for your chosen leader.[2] I believe with all of my heart that if we get on our knees and regularly lift up our elected officials in prayer, God will change their hearts and once again we will be a nation under God, submitted to His leadership.

I hope you'll allow me to relate a personal example of the type of stresses that occur to those in leadership positions. I was having lunch with a friend at a restaurant one day. Now I have very sensitive teeth, and I don't like ice hitting them because it hurts, so I always order water with a straw. About a week later I received a letter from a woman who wrote, "Mrs. Dobson, I recognized you in a restaurant. I noticed that you ordered water with a straw." She implied in her note, "What was I afraid of? Was I afraid of AIDS?"

When you are in a leadership position, people notice the strangest things. Everything is under scrutiny—every word you say, everything your kids do, even what kind of *toothpaste* you use! I can't imagine why people pick at you and criticize you and watch everything you do, but when God places you in a visible position, they just do. It can be very stressful at times. I just want to say that this "celebrity" business is an illusion. People in visible positions have the same hurts as you do, they experience the same pain as you do. They have the same needs, the same joys. They are not any different; they're just ordinary people.

Our officials in local, state, and national positions are husbands, wives, dads and moms, neighbors and friends. We need to be lifting them up in prayer. I want to encourage you to consider adopting a leader for one year and letting him or her know that instead of sending notes of criticism to them, you are going to be sending notes of encouragement, notes telling them that you are praying for them and that you care for them and their families.

As we go to prayer, I want you to think about the leaders in your city. It could be your mayor; it could be a city council member or a state senator—whomever God brings to your mind. Think about the leaders on the national level as well. Let's lift them up in prayer. Before we begin, in your own heart could you silently pray, "Lord, is there a leader in my community, in my state, or on a national level that I could adopt for one year?" See if the Lord doesn't bring someone to your mind.

Physical Aspects of Fasting

Many of you have written to me or called the fasting telephone line with questions regarding the physical aspects of fasting. As you know, I am not a medical doctor and strongly recommend that if you have physical problems or experience them while fasting, you should seek medical advice.

T*he Coming Revival* gave a call for two million believers to undertake a forty-day fast to pray for spiritual revival for America and the world and for the fulfillment of the Great Commission. Guidelines for fasting were offered as well as a directive by a medical doctor. Many questions have come to my attention since its publication, which I will attempt to address. However, I also recommend researching the numerous books written by experts on the physical aspects of fasting. (Refer to the Resources section at the back of this book.)

My emphasis is extended juice-fasting only, and I strongly warn against attempting a forty-day, water-only fast apart from medical supervision. Water-only fasts that last for more than several days need to be undertaken with *complete rest* and *under medical supervision* because of the extreme danger of over-toxification, breakdown of vital body tissues, and loss of electrolytes.

This call to fasting is for spiritual reasons, to seek after God by de-emphasizing the needs of the body and elevating the needs of the spirit. At the same time, I recognize the physical benefits of fasting. Dr. James and Phyllis Balch write in *Prescription for Nutritional Healing:*

> Fasting can help reverse the aging process, and if we use it correctly, we will live longer, happier lives...You can fight off illness and the degenerative diseases so common in this chemically polluted environment we live in...You heal faster, give your organs a rest, clean your liver and kidneys, purify your blood, cleanse your colon, lose unnecessary weight, get rid of toxin build-up in tissues, clear the eyes and tongue, cleanse the breath, and lose excess water.[1]

With a juice fast, most of us can continue fairly normal work patterns. The nutrients we need will be supplied by a variety of juices from fruits and vegetables. The amount of juices you need each day will depend on your daily exertions, size, and metabolism. Christian nutritionist Pamela Smith recommends drinking "twelve ounces of juice at your meal times and six ounces every two hours between meals, along with up to two to three quarts of water spread evenly throughout the day...Drink lukewarm or cool water throughout the day and exercise moderately."[2]

Varying the types of juices you drink during the day will assure that you will receive the nutrients your body needs. Vegetable juices will supply the electrolytes necessary for proper heart functions. Fresh-squeezed juices are recommended. Any store-bought juice should be free of sugar (corn syrup, etc.) and salt. Acidic juices, such as orange or tomato, will be better tolerated if they are half juice, half water. Herbal teas and a pure vegetable broth (oil- and salt-free) can also be part of the daily intake.

The juices, herbal teas, and vegetable broth will pass through the stomach without starting the digestive system and will keep your body burning the low-grade stored fat, so you will not feel hungry. Any product containing protein or fat, such as milk or soy-based drinks, will restart digestion and you will again feel hunger pangs.

If you have not fasted before, begin with a one-day fast and gradually increase to a ten-day fast. After a ten-day fast, the body has cleansed itself from many toxins. This process also will make you aware of what to expect and calm many of the fears of fasting.

The first three days are the most difficult regarding hunger pangs. Your body is shifting from using the food in the stomach (which lasts three days) to consuming stored fats. During that time, many have found that taking psyllium bulk or seed capsules[3] helps eliminate hunger pangs and also aids in cleansing the body. Several capsules can be taken throughout the day with plenty of water. Silymarin tablets protect and enhance cleansing of the liver.

Fasting Discomfort

It is normal to feel colder than usual, to experience bad breath and heightened body odor, changes in elimination (constipation or diarrhea), light-headedness, changes in sleeping and dreaming patterns, or aches and pains. A white-coated tongue at the beginning of a fast is part of the body's pattern of throwing off toxins.

After the first two weeks of a fast, many of these symptoms subside. Continuing aches in a certain area of the body usually means elimination of fatty tissue is going on in that area, which is not harmful. However, any extensive pain should be examined immediately. **You should stop fasting if you are experiencing severe pain or swelling.**

Most people can complete a juice fast without any unusual problems. When there are uncomfortable times, thank the Lord for the opportunity to cleanse the physical body as our spirit is cleansed. During a long fast, many people are temporarily freed from arthritis and other constant pains they normally experience.

Headaches or stomach aches may be a result of salt, sugar, or caffeine withdrawal. Eliminating these items from your diet prior to fasting is the best way to avoid these pains. Lower back pain may indicate that you are dehydrating and need to drink more fluids. Alfalfa tablets will control bad breath and help to cleanse the system. Two tablets at a time can be taken several times a day.

Light-headedness can be controlled by getting up from bed or stooping positions slowly to keep the blood pressure stable. Lie down if you feel faint. Congestion occurs when the body is eliminating toxins. Elimination of loose, mucous, or dark stools is no cause for alarm and is part of the cleansing. Resting and staying warm will help the body through rough times.

If you are overly concerned about what is happening in your body, if there is severe discomfort, or if you feel that you are jeopardizing your health, break your fast *slowly* using the guidelines that follow. You may not be able to do an extended forty-day fast for physical reasons. God honors fasting for short amounts of time, one or two days a week, or other kinds of fasts as well. It's not the number of days that is important; it is the act of humbling ourselves in fasting before the Lord. After three personal forty-day fasts (1994, 1995, 1996), I strongly recommend that every believer who is physically healthy pray and work for at least one forty-day fast. Nothing that I have ever experienced results in a greater intimacy with God if followed with proper motive to seek God's face.

Act responsibly regarding your health while fasting. Most people feel better than they do normally, although their daily strength is usually diminished.

Breaking Your Fast

All the experts agree that this is the critical phase of fasting. When your body has been in the resting mode, your stomach shrinks and your intestines become idle, so solid food must be introduced very slowly to avoid any fatal conditions such as kidney failure or bursting intestines. *After a forty-day fast, take at least seven days before returning to*

eating meats or fats. There may be a desire to gorge on long-missed
foods, but it is very, very dangerous to do so.

Dr. Paul Bragg and his daughter Patricia have conduct-
ed fasting clinics for many years. Their book *The Miracle of*
Fasting gives a specific daily food plan for breaking a
seven-day fast that could be adapted and stretched out over
several more days for those completing a forty-day fast.

Around 5 o'clock of the 7th day of the fast, peel
four or five medium-sized tomatoes, cut them up,
bring them to a boil and then turn off the heat, and
when they are cool enough to eat, have as many as you
desire.

On the morning of the 8th day, you are to have a
salad of grated carrots and grated cabbage, with half
an orange squeezed over it. After your salad, you may
have a bowl of steamed greens and peeled tomatoes
(spinach, Swiss chard, or mustard greens). Bring the
greens to a boil, then turn off the heat. With your
greens, you may eat two slices of 100-percent whole-
wheat bread which has been toasted until it is thor-
oughly dry—this is called "Melba toast." After it has
cooled, the toast should be so dry that it would pow-
der if you squeezed it in the palm of your hand. As I
have stated, this first food should be in the morning.
During the day, you may have all the distilled water
you wish to drink.

For dinner, you may have a salad of grated carrots,
chopped celery and cabbage, with orange juice for
dressing. This will be followed by two cooked vegetables, one such as spinach, kale, chard, or mustard
greens, and one such as string beans, carrots, steamed
celery, okra, or squash. You may have two pieces of
whole-grain "Melba toast." These meals are not to con-
tain oils of any kind.

On the morning of the 9th day, you may have a
dish of any kind of fresh fruit, such as banana, pineap-
ple, orange, sliced grapefruit, or sliced apples. You

may sprinkle this with two tablespoonsful of raw wheat germ, and sweeten it with honey, but not over one tablespoonful. At noon you may have a salad of grated carrots, cabbage, and celery, with one cooked vegetable and one slice of "Melba toast." At dinner you may have a salad dish of lettuce, watercress, parsley and tomatoes, and two cooked vegetables.[4]

Most experts agree that breaking a fast with vegetables, either steamed or raw, is best. Go along with your smaller stomach and eat lightly. Stop before you feel full. Stay away from starches like pastas, potatoes, rice, or bread, except for the "Melba toast," for a least a week. Also avoid meats, dairy products, and any fats or oils for at least a week, then reintroduce them very slowly and in small amounts.

The weight you lose during a fast usually returns gradually after resuming normal eating. However, one person who fasted reports the following:

> When I finished my forty-day fast, no weight came back on for a whole year. If you will stay on a "Daniel" fast for several weeks after a juice fast, you will not gain weight: vegetables and fruit and water; no breads, no grains, no fats, no meats—just vegetables and fruit. After that, go back very, very gradually to adding anything else in your diet, and the weight will not come back.

After the fast, resist the urge to rush into your normal schedule. The body still is working at a slower level and your metabolism may be sluggish as you begin eating. That is normal and will gradually increase.

These are suggestions to answer some of the basic questions you may have about fasting. Medical advice regarding special conditions should be procured from your doctor. Those who have specific conditions such as diabetes or hypoglycemia, or are pregnant, would be well-advised not to fast.

Initiating a Corporate Fast

To offer assistance to those who would like to organize a corporate fast, I have listed the following methods that have come to our attention. Many of the citywide and churchwide efforts grew out of already established pastors' gatherings. They, in turn, motivated their congregations and used contacts to obtain facilities, media, music, and other arrangements.

Citywide Efforts

Melinda Fuschetto organized a fasting effort in Raleigh, North Carolina. She comments on the free advertising she received:

> As you might have guessed, there were no funds available to advertise the way we would have liked to. We sent out Public Service Announcements to eight newspapers, six Christian radio stations, and three TV stations. I made two thirty-second commercials that aired on a Raleigh Cable TV Christian program that airs six days a week. Posters and flyers went out to the nine Christian bookstores in the Raleigh/Durham area. Hundreds of flyers were taken in the first few days.

A citywide fast was organized by several of the pastors in Katy, Texas. They were able to receive the backing of the mayor and city council. The following proclamation and advertising were printed in the local newspaper:

City of Katy

PROCLAMATION
BY THE
MAYOR OF THE CITY OF KATY, TEXAS

HUB CITY OF THREE COUNTIES

TO ALL TO WHOM THESE PRESENTS SHALL COME:

WHEREAS,   A 40 day period of Prayer and Fasting is intended to unite the people of Katy in an effort to Strengthen the spiritual foundations of our community; and,

WHEREAS,   Katy has always been a City of strong Judeo - Christian values; and,

WHEREAS,   There is concern that the loss of spiritual foundation in a community will eventually devastate a City as it can an individual; and,

WHEREAS,   There has been a noble effort on the part of Katy Independent School District Trustees to encourage the teaching of basic traditional values such as respect, patriotism, patience, self-discipline, etc., to our children; and,

WHEREAS,   There is strong evidence of spiritual awakening taking place among some cities and communities across America;

NOW THEREFORE, I, M. H. "Hank" Schmidt, Jr., Mayor of the City of Katy, with the support of the Katy City Council, do hereby proclaim May 2 through June 10, 1996, as

"40 DAYS OF PRAYER AND FASTING" in Katy

and call upon all of our citizens to participate in this 40 day event at the safe and spiritual level at which they choose.

WITNESS my hand and the Seal of the City of Katy, Texas, this the 22 day of April, 1996.

_____
Mayor

ATTEST:

_____
City Secretary

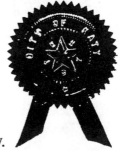

May 2 - June 10
Citizens of Katy, let us pray together for God to renew and strengthen our beloved community.
(Pastors Prayer Fellowship)

A Call
To Prayer
And Fasting

Mayor Hank Schmidt has issued a proclamation, urging the citizens of Katy to pray and fast for 40 days in behalf of our community.

During these days (May 2 - June 10), would you join with our neighbors, fellow employees, school-mates, etc in asking God to Spiritually renew our city?

City-wide prayer sessions will be held

May 15 (Wednesday Night)
First United Methodist Church
7:00 - 7:40 P.M.
May 26 (Sunday Night)
7:00 - 7:40 P.M.
Pastor's Prayer Fellowship

A list of "Levels of Participation" was also printed in the Katy newspaper:

Prayer

1. Attend weekly prayer meetings held in each church or temple.
2. Attend community prayer meetings which will be hosted interdenominationally during this period.
3. Businessmen and women are encouraged to gather for periods of prayer on behalf of the city.
4. Social clubs and other organizations are encouraged to pray for Katy.
5. Cottage prayer meetings are encouraged to meet in homes throughout the communities as hosts invite neighbors in.
6. Students at schools may find time to voluntarily pray together when it will not disturb daily classes and schedules.

Fasting

1. Full forty days
2. One week
3. One full day each week for six weeks
4. One meal a day for forty days
5. If health prevents fasting food, one might choose to fast some other pleasures (TV, leisure activities, etc.)

Please consult your physician before attempting any fast. A forty-day fast would require consumption of water and juice.

Participants in citywide fasts often rotated their meeting place to different participating churches to maintain inclusiveness. If space was prohibitive, alternating pastors would lead at the largest building available. Worship styles were varied as well. Maintaining an orderly yet Spirit-led meeting allowed everyone to enjoy participation. (See a list of guidelines in Chapter 4, "Revival Is Coming!")

Churchwide Efforts

Pastor Brian Warner prepared his church for fasting by giving four messages on fasting prior to the forty days. The church bulletin featured a section on fasting news and support. People were given instruction about fasting and were also directed to published information. A fasting and prayer support group met every Friday evening that ministered to those fasting and also prayed for the church, city, and nation. Pastor Warner notes that the support group was very helpful.

Roy Mansfield of Manhattan Bible Church, New York City, prepared a spiral bound booklet to lead the congregation in a fasting day each month. *Guide for a Day of Prayer and Fasting* offered information on preparing for a fast day, an hour-specific prayer guide, information on each item on the prayer list, Scripture verses and teaching, personal attributes for the believer, the attributes of God, and pages for recording prayers and noting the way God is leading.

The Department of Evangelism and Church Growth of the Wesleyan Church in Indianapolis, Indiana, makes available a packet of sample materials for each of its member churches for an annual forty-day emphasis on fasting and prayer. Built around an annual theme, the program materials include sermon resources, worship and drama resources, personal spiritual journal, daily prayer calendar, theme poster, prayer reminders, clip art, small group guides, and theme-related books. Materials are available from the Wesleyan Publishing House (800-493-7539).

Campus Crusade for Christ's Fasting & Prayer Office is soliciting news and testimonies about fasting and prayer activities for their Web page and other publications. Please E-mail your testimony to fasting&prayer@ccci.org or mail it to the Fasting & Prayer Office, Campus Crusade for Christ, 100 Sunport Lane #2100, Orlando, FL 32809-7871. The Internet address is www.ccci.org/fasting-prayer97.

The Purposes of Fasting with Prayer

1. To honor God (Matthew 6:16–18; Zechariah 7:5; Luke 2:37; Acts 13:2).

2. To humble ourselves before God (Ezra 8:21; Psalm 69:10; Isaiah 58:3) in order to experience more grace (1 Peter 5:5) and God's intimate presence (Isaiah 57:15; 58:6–9).

3. To mourn over personal sin and failure (1 Samuel 7:6; Nehemiah 9:1,2).

4. To mourn over the sins of the church, nation, and world (1 Samuel 7:6; Nehemiah 9:1,2).

5. To seek grace for a new task, for the work God has sent us to do, and to reaffirm our consecration to God (Matthew 4:2).

6. To seek God by drawing near to him and persisting in prayer against opposing spiritual forces (Judges 20:26; Ezra 8:21,23,31; Jeremiah 29:12–14; Joel 2:12; Luke 18:3; Acts 9:10–19).

7. To show repentance and so make a way for God to change his declared intentions of judgment (2 Samuel 12:16,22; 1 Kings 21:27–29; Jeremiah 18:7,8; Joel 2:12–14; Jonah 3:5,10).

8. To save people from bondage to evil (Isaiah 58:6; Matthew 17:14–21; Luke 4:1).

9. To gain revelation and wisdom concerning God's will (Isaiah 58:5,6,11; Daniel 9:3,21,22; Acts 13:2,3).

10. To open the way for the outpouring of the Spirit and Christ's return to earth for His people (Matthew 9:15; 25:6; John 14:3).

Fasting in This Age

1. Is a sign of the believer's longing for the Lord's return.
2. Is a preparation for Christ's coming.
3. Is a mourning of Christ's absence.
4. Is a sign of sorrow for the sin and decay of the world.

Used with permission. From the *Full Life Study Bible—New International Version*, pp. 1415, 1422. Copyrighted by Life Publishers International, Springfield, MO, 1992.

Proud Spirits and Humble Hearts

Nancy Leigh DeMoss contrasts characteristics of proud, unbroken people who are resistant to the call of God on their lives with the qualities of broken, humble people who have experienced God's revival. Read each item on the list as you ask God to reveal which characteristics of a proud spirit He finds in your life. Confess these to Him, then ask Him to restore the corresponding quality of a broken, humble spirit in you.

Proud, Unbroken People	Humble, Broken People
Focus on the failure of others	Overwhelmed with a sense of their own spiritual need
Self-righteous; have a critical, fault-finding spirit; look at their own life/faults through a telescope but at others with a microscope	Compassionate; forgiving; look for the best in others
Look down on others	Esteem all others better than self
Independent/self-sufficient spirit	Dependent spirit; recognize need for others
Maintain control; must be their way	Surrender control
Have to prove that they are right	Willing to yield the right to be right
Claim rights	Yield rights

Proud, Unbroken People	Humble, Broken People
Demanding spirit	Giving spirit
Desire to be served	Motivated to serve others
Desire for self-advancement	Desire to promote others
Driven to be recognized/appreciated	Sense of unworthiness; thrilled to be used at all; eager for others to get credit
Wounded when others are promoted	Rejoice when others are lifted up and they are over-looked
"The ministry is privileged to have me."	"I don't deserve to serve in this ministry."
Think of what they can do for God	Know that they have nothing to offer God
Feel confident in how much they know	Humbled by how much they have to learn
Self-conscious	Not concerned with self at all
Keep people at arm's length	Risk getting close to others; willing to take the risk of loving intimately
Quick to blame others	Accept personal responsibility—can see where they are wrong
Unapproachable	"Easy to be entreated"
Defensive when criticized	Receive criticism with a humble, open heart
Concerned with being "respectable"	Concerned with being real
Concerned with what others think	All that matters is what God knows
Work to maintain image/protect reputation	Die to own reputation

Proud, Unbroken People	Humble, Broken People
Find it difficult to share their spiritual needs with others	Willing to be open and transparent with others
Want to be sure nobody finds out about their sin	Willing to be exposed (once broken, they don't care who knows—nothing to lose)
Have a hard time saying, "I was wrong; will you please forgive me?"	Quick to admit failure and seek forgiveness
When confessing sin, deal in generalities	Deal in specifics
Concerned about the consequences of their sins	Grieved over the cause or root of their sins
Remorseful over their sin— got caught/found out	Repentant over sin (forsake it)
When there is a misunder-standing or conflict, wait for the other to come and ask forgiveness	Take the initiative to be rec-onciled; see if they can get to the cross first!
Compare themselves with others and feel deserving of honor	Compare themselves to the holiness of God and feel desperate need for mercy
Don't think they have anything to repent of	Continual heart attitude of repentance
Don't think they need revival (think everybody else does)	Continually sense their need for a fresh infilling of the Holy Spirit

Notes

Chapter 2

1. C. S. Lewis, *Letters to an American Lady*, William B. Eerdman's Publishing Company, Grand Rapids, p. 49.

Chapter 3

1. Appendix D, "Initiating a Corporate Fast," suggests practical ways in which groups have organized a large-scale effort.
2. Part of Nancy's address is reprinted in Appendix G, "Proud Spirits and Humble Hearts."
3. J. Doug Stringer, "It's Time, Houston!" *November 1996 Update,* Turning Point Ministries, International, Houston, Texas, p. 2.
4. J. Doug Stringer, "Houston's Date With Destiny" *Prayer Mountain Update,* December 1996, p. 4.
5. Claire Greiner, "Houston's Prayer Mountain: 40 Days in Review," p. 1
6. Greiner, p. 2.
7. The *First Friday* newsletter is available through Intercessors For America, P.O. Box 4477, Leesburg, VA 20177.
8. The complete talk by Nancy Leigh DeMoss is available on cassette through Campus Crusade Direct, (800) 729-4351.
9. You can contact the Fasting & Prayer Chain International at 94-941 Kau'Olu Place #703, Waipahu, HI 96797. Phone (808) 671-2555; fax (808) 677-2351.

Chapter 4

1. Bill Bright, *The Coming Revival,* NewLife Publications, p. 69.
2. Karen Hill, "West Texas Revival," *Evangelism Today,* Volume 3, 1996, p. 6.
3. Hill, p. 6.
4. For more information on how to share your faith and disciple others, see my book *Witnessing Without Fear.* Ordering information is given in the Resources section at the back of this book.

Appendix C

1. Dr. James Dobson of Focus on the Family.
2. For information, contact the National Day of Prayer Task Force, P.O. Box 15616, Colorado Springs, CO 80935-5616; (719) 531-3379.

Appendix D

1. Balch, James F. and Phyllis A., *Prescription for Nutritional Healing*, Avery Publishing Group, Inc., p. 325.
2. Smith, Pamela, "Guidelines for Fasting," *Charisma*, January 1996.
3. "Perfect 7" made by Agape Health Products works well and does not interfere with fasting. It can be found in many health food stores.
4. Bragg, Paul C. and Patricia, *The Miracle of Fasting*, Health Science, p. 75.

Resources for
Further Reading

Avant, John; McDow, Malcolm; and Reid, Alvin. *Revival!* Nashville, TN: Broadman & Holman Publishers, 1996.

Balch, James F. and Phyllis. *Prescription for Nutritional Healing.* Garden City, NY: Avery Publishing Group, Inc., 1990.

Beall, James Lee. *The Adventure of Fasting.* Old Tappan, NJ: Fleming H. Revell, Co., 1974.

Blackaby, Henry T., and King, Claude V. *Experiencing God.* Nashville, TN: Broadman & Holman Publishers, 1994.

Blackaby, Henry T., and King, Claude V. *Fresh Encounter.* Nashville, TN: Broadman & Holman Publishers, 1996.

Bragg, Paul C. and Patricia. *The Miracle of Fasting.* Santa Barbara, CA: Health Science, 1987.

Bright, Bill. *The Christian and Prayer.* Orlando, FL: NewLife Publications, 1994.

Bright, Bill. *The Coming Revival.* Orlando, FL: NewLife Publications, 1995.

Bright, Bill. *How to Lead a Successful Fasting & Prayer Gathering.* Orlando, FL: NewLife Publications, 1995.

Bright, Bill. *Seven Basic Steps to Successful Fasting & Prayer.* Orlando, FL: NewLife Publications, 1995.

Bright, Vonette, & Jennings, B. *Unleashing the Power of Prayer.* Chicago: Moody Press, 1989.

Brown, Steve. *Approaching God.* Nashville, TN: Moorings, 1996.

Bryant, David. *Concerts of Prayer.* Ventura, CA: Regal Books, 1988.

Bueno, Lee. *Fast Your Way to Health.* Springdale, PA: Whitaker House, 1991.

Christensen, Evelyn. *"Lord, Change Me!"* Wheaton, IL: Victor Books, 1977.

Eastman, Dick. *The Jericho Hour.* Lake Mary, FL: Creation House, 1994.

Eastman, Dick. *Love On Its Knees.* Fairfax, VA: Chosen Books, 1989.

Edwards, Brian H. *Revival!* Durham, England: Evangelical Press, 1990.

Elliot, Elisabeth. *Discipline: The Glad Surrender.* Old Tappan, NJ: Fleming H. Revell, 1982.

Floyd, Ronnie W. *God's Gateway to Supernatural Power.* Nashville, TN: Sunday School Board of the Southern Baptist Convention, 1996.

Floyd, Ronnie W. *The Meaning of a Man.* Nashville, TN: Broadman & Holman, 1996.

Floyd, Ronnie W. *The Power of Prayer and Fasting.* Nashville, TN: Broadman & Holman, 1997.

Foster, Richard J. *Prayer.* San Francisco: Harper San-Francisco, 1992.

Green, Paul A. *Churches on Fire.* Concerts of Prayer, 1994.

Grubb, Norman. *Rees Howells, Intercessor.* Fort Washington, PA: Christian Literature Crusade, 1952.

Lewis, C. S. *Letters to Malcolm Chiefly on Prayer.* Harcourt Brace Jovanovich Publishers, 1963.

Lindsay, Gordon. *Prayer & Fasting.* Dallas: Christ for the Nations, Inc., 1994.

Lloyd-Jones, Martyn. *Revival.* Wheaton, IL: Crossway Books, 1987.

Nelson, Alan E. *Broken in the Right Place.* Nashville, TN: Thomas Nelson Publishers, 1994.

Omartian, Stormie. *Greater Health God's Way.* Chatsworth, CA: Sparrow Press, 1984.

Packer, J. I. *A Quest for Godliness.* Wheaton, IL: Crossway Books, 1990.

Prince, Derek. *Fasting.* Springdale, PA: Whitaker House, 1986.

Prince, Derek. *Shaping History Through Prayer and Fasting.* Old Tappan, NJ: Fleming H. Revell Co., 1973.

Ravenhill, Leonard. *Why Revival Tarries.* Minneapolis: Bethany House Publishers, 1986.

Ruibal, Julio. *Fasting* video available through Ruibal Foundation, P.O. Box 1830, Pinellas Park, FL 34664-1830.

Russell, Rex. *What the Bible Says About Healthy Living.* Ventura, CA: Regal Books, 1996.

Sheets, Dutch. *Intercessory Prayer: Discover How Your Prayers Can Move Heaven & Earth.* Ventura, CA: Regal Books, 1996.

Smith, Alice. *Beyond the Veil.* Houston: SpiriTruth Publishing Company, 1996.

Smith, Alice. *Power Praying: Instruction on Prayer & Fasting.* Houston: SpiriTruth Publishing Company, 1996.

Towns, Elmer L. *Fasting for Spiritual Breakthrough.* Ventura, CA: Regal Books, 1996.

Tirabassi, Becky. *Wild Things Happen When I Pray.* Grand Rapids, MI: Zondervan, 1994.

Wagner, C. Peter. *Churches That Pray.* Ventura, CA: Regal Books, 1993.

Wallis, Arthur. *God's Chosen Fast.* Fort Washington, PA: Christian Literature Crusade, 1968.

Whitney, Donald S. *Spiritual Disciplines for the Christian Life.* Colorado Springs, CO: NavPress, 1991.

Yancey, Philip. *The Jesus I Never Knew.* Grand Rapids, MI: Zondervan Publishing House, 1995.

Our nation is in a moral free-fall and the Church for the most part is spiritually impotent. What can we do to stop the tragic decline? This book gives the startling answer! Easy-to-read. The thoughts are fresh. The challenge is compelling. (224 pp., $9.99)

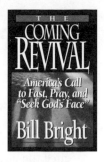

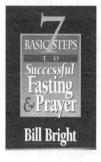

This handy reference guide to fasting and prayer available alone or as a companion to *The Coming Revival*. Contains instructions on how to begin, maintain, and break your fast with results. (24 pp., $.99)

Now, for the first time, you can lead a fasting and prayer gathering in your small group or in your church or community. Step-by-step instructions on how to develop a leadership team and conduct the gathering. (48 pp., $4.99)

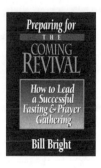

How You Can Pray With Confidence. Based on life-changing biblical truths, this booklet provides practical and powerful steps to deeper communion with God. Part of the Transferable Concepts series. (64 pp., $1.99)

How You Can Be Filled With the Holy Spirit. This time-tested booklet provides insight on the dynamic process of being filled with the Holy Spirit. This booklet shows how to live with a new dimension of happiness and joy every day. Part of the Transferable Concepts series. (64 pp., $1.99)

How You Can Walk in the Spirit. This booklet teaches Christians how to face real-life problems and disappointments in the power of the Holy Spirit and enables you to be victorious over temptation. Part of the Transferable Concepts series. (64 pp., $1.99)

Response Form

☐ I have received Jesus Christ as my Savior and Lord as a result of reading this book.

☐ I am a new Christian and want to know Christ better and experience the abundant Christian life.

☐ I want to be one of the two million people who will join you in forty days of fasting and prayer for revival.

☐ I have completed an extended or forty-day fast with prayer and am enclosing my written testimony to encourage and bless others.

☐ Please send me **free** information on staff and ministry opportunities with Campus Crusade for Christ.

☐ Please send me **free** information about other books, booklets, audio cassettes, and videos by Bill and Vonette Bright.

NAME_____

ADDRESS_____

CITY _____ STATE _____ ZIP _____

COUNTRY _____

Please check the appropriate box(es), clip, and mail this form in an envelope to:

> Dr. Bill Bright
> Campus Crusade for Christ
> P.O. Box 593684
> Orlando, FL 62859-3684

You may also fax your response to (407) 826-2149 or send E-mail to:

> CompuServe: 74114,1206
> Internet: newlife@magicnet.net

This and other fine products from NewLife Publications are available from your favorite bookseller or by calling **(800) 235-7255** *(within U.S.) or* **(407) 826-2145** *(outside U.S.).*